Mahāmudrā and Atiyoga

Emerging Perceptions in Buddhist Studies
(ISSN 0971-9512)

1-2. An Encyclopaedia of Buddhist Deities, Demigods, Godlings, Saints & Demons — with Special Focus on Iconographic Attributes; by Fredrick W. Bunce. 2 Vols. (ISBN 81-246-0020-1; set)

3. Buddhism in Karnataka; by R.C. Hiremath; with a foreword by H.H. the Dalai Lama (ISBN 81-246-0013-9)

4-5. Pāli Language and Literature: A Systematic Survey and Historical Study; by Kanai Lal Hazra. 2 Vols. (ISBN 81-246-0004-X; set)

6. Maṇḍala and Landscape; by A.W. Macdonald (ISBN 81-246-0060-0)

7. The Future Buddha Maitreya: An Iconological Study; by Inchang Kim (ISBN 81-246-0082-1)

8. Absence of the Buddha Image in Early Buddhist Art; by Kanoko Tanaka (ISBN 81-246-0090-2)

9. A Few Facts About Buddhism; by Gunnar Gällmo (ISBN 81-246-0099-6)

10. Buddhist Theory of Meaning and Literary Analysis; by Rajnish K. Mishra (ISBN 81-246-0118-6)

11. Buddhism as/in Performance; Analysis of Meditation and Theatrical Practice; by David E.R. George (ISBN 81-246-0123-2)

12. Buddhist Tantra and Buddhist Art; by T.N. Mishra (ISBN 81-246-0141-0)

13. Buddhist Art in India and Sri Lanka: 3rd Century BC to 6th Century AD — A Critical Study; by Virender Kumar Dabral (ISBN 81-246-0162-3)

14. The Tibetan Iconography of Buddhas, Bodhisattvas and Other Deities — A Unique Pantheon; by Lokesh Chandra & Fredrick W. Bunce (ISBN 81-246-0178-X)

15. The Dalai Lamas — The Institution and Its History by Ardy Verhaegen; (ISBN 81-246-0202-6)

16. The Tibetan Tāntric Vision; by Krishna Ghosh Della Santina (ISBN 81-246-0227-1)

17. The Buddhist Art of Kauśāmbī; by Aruna Tripathi: From 300 BC to AD 550 (ISBN 81-246-0226-3)

18. Mahāmudrā and Atiyoga; by Giuseppe Baroetto; Translated from Italian into English by Andrew Lukianowicz (ISBN 81-246-0322-7)

19. Theravāda Buddhist Devotionalism in Ceylon, Burma and Thailand; by V.V.S. Saibaba (ISBN 81-246-0327-8)

20. Faith and Devotion in Theravāda Buddhism; by V.V.S. Saibaba (ISBN 81-246-0329-4)

Emerging Perceptions in Buddhist Studies, no. 18

Mahāmudrā and Atiyoga

by
Giuseppe Baroetto

Translated from Italian into English by
Andrew Lukianowicz

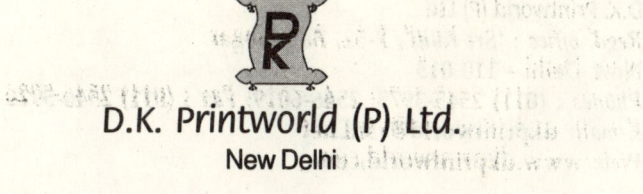

D.K. Printworld (P) Ltd.
New Delhi

Cataloging in Publication Data — DK
[Courtesy: D.K. Agencies (P) Ltd. <docinfo@dkagencies.com>]

Baroetto, Giuseppe, 1959-
   Mahāmudrā and Atiyoga / by Giuseppe Baroetto; translated from Italian into English by Andrew Lukianowicz.
   p. 23 cm. — (Emerging perceptions in Buddhist studies; no. 18)
   Appendices in Tibetan (roman)
   ISBN 8124603227

   1. Mahāmudrā (Tantric rite). 2. Rdzogs-chen (Rñiṅ-ma-pa). 3. Tantric Buddhism — Rituals. 4. Yoga — Tantric Buddhism. 5. Tantric Buddhism.
   I. Title. II. Series: Emerging perceptions in Buddhist studies ; no. 18.

DDC 294.392 5   21

ISBN 81-246-0322-7
First Published in India in 2005
© Authors

All rights reserved. No part of this publication may be reproduced or transmitted in any form or by any means, electronic or mechanical, including photocopying, recording, or any information storage or retrieval system, without prior written permission of the copyright holders, indicated above.

Published and printed by:
D.K. Printworld (P) Ltd.
Regd. office : *'Sri Kunj'*, F-52, Bali Nagar
New Delhi - 110 015
Phones : (011) 2545-3975; 2546-6019; *Fax* : (011) 2546-5926
E-mail: dkprintworld@vsnl.net
Web: www.dkprintworld.com

Prologue

THIS volume comprises translations, commentaries and transliteration of some ancient Tibetan texts, significant documents of the wisdom heritage handed down in the "Land of Snow."

In the following pages, the academic training and philosophical interest that have formed and motivated my research into Tibet's religious traditions encounter the personal experiences of two Lamas, who have marked a crucial change in my approach to Indo-Tibetan studies.

Mahāmudrā and *Atiyoga* are particular forms of Buddhist spirituality that, although differentiated by distinct historical lineages, meet in the same radical essentiality where human beings, transcending their dividing attitudes, find themselves truly free in the single reality that has always unified them all.

Contents

Prologue	v
I. MAHĀMUDRĀ	1
1. Premise	3
2. Advice on the Great Seal	5
3. Commentary	10
4. The Treasury of Hymns	36
5. Commentary	38
II. ATIYOGA	49
1. Premise	51
2. The Introduction to Awareness	54
3. Commentary	69
III. APPENDICES	129
(Transliteration of the Tibetan texts)	
Appendix 1 — *Phyag rgya chen po'i man ngag*	131
Appendix 2 — *Do ha mdzod ces bya ba/*	137
Appendix 3 — *:Zab chos zhi khro Dgongs pa rang grol las:*	139
Appendix 4 — *Kun byed rgyal po*	162
Index	181

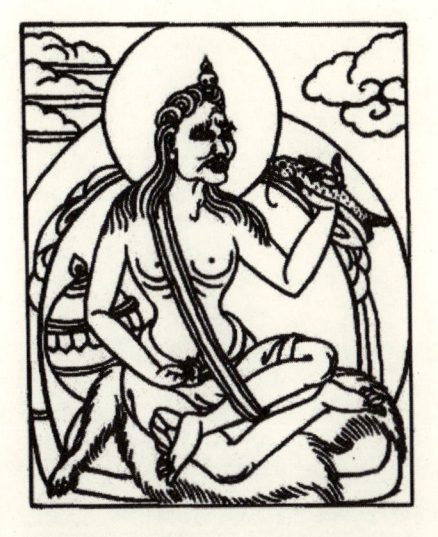

Tilopa (Courtesy: www.buddhanet.net)

PART I
MAHĀMUDRĀ

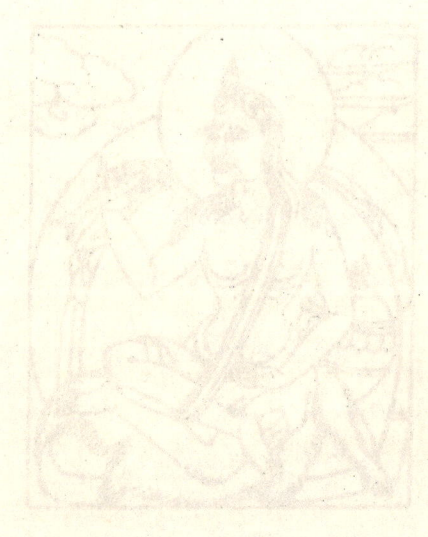

1. Premise

THE two texts translated here from the Tibetan are ascribed to Tilopa (928-1009),[1] the celebrated Indian mystic, famous above all for having initiated the learned master Nāropa (956-1040) into the ultimate meaning of a teaching known in Sanskrit as *Mahāmudrā*, the "Great Seal." This spirituality is considered by Tibetan teachers to be the essence of both the short (*gseng lam*) or instantaneous path (*cig car ba*), free of any form of meditation or support, and the final instructions that conclude the gradual (*rim gyis pa*) common and esoteric paths of Buddhist doctrines based on the Sūtras and Tantras respectively.[2]

The commentary is a transcription of the oral instructions I received in October 1989 from a Tibetan teacher in Nepal at Swayambhunath, near Kathmandu. At that time, I was

---

1. My translation is based on the Tibetan versions, published in *Do ha mdzod brgyad*, Tashijong, Palampur (India), 1973: *Phyag rgya chen po'i man ngag (Mahāmudrā-upadeśa)*, ff. 14b-18a = A; *Do ha mdzod ces bya ba (Dohakośanāma)*, ff. 11a-12a. Concerning the former, in my notes I have also taken into account the variants present in Kong sprul Blo gros mtha' yas' edition: *gDams ngag mdzod*, Delhi, 1971, vol. V, pp. 33-36 = B; Cf. Francis Tiso and Fabrizio Torricelli, "The Tibetan Text of Tilopa's *Mahāmudropadeśa*," *East and West*, XLI, 1991, pp. 205-29.

2. On the distinction between the two paths, see Takpo Tashi Namgyal, *Mahāmudrā — The Quintessence of Mind and Meditation*, Boston & London, 1986, pp. 101, 110-18, 123-25.

translating the two texts by Tilopa from their Tibetan versions, however without having previously requested the authorization and instructions from a preceptor of those teachings, as required by the tradition.

On finishing my circumambulation of the *stūpa*, I saw standing still before me an elderly Tibetan monk, staring at me. I nodded a greeting and he smiled, singing: "I pay homage to the teacher of the Great Seal."

After a few seconds of amazement and confusion, I realized that he had penetrated my presumptuousness. Evidently, he was a teacher of what I was laboriously trying to understand with my intellect. I immediately thought of asking the Lama whether he would be willing to explain the meaning of the Great Seal to me, but, without even giving me time to speak, he told me: "I am Lhündrup Tenzin. You have met me because you were seeking me. If you want the transmission and explanation of Tilopa's advice, then follow me." So I did.

The Lama entered a temple, sat on the ground, and after bidding me do the same he started giving the "oral transmission" of the Tibetan texts, chanting them by heart with a slow, harmonious melody. Immediately afterwards he started his commentary, emphasizing the most meaningful and essential aspects with language that was simple and, at the same time, clear and precise. I noticed that his words flowed unhurriedly, intermitted by long pauses, probably intended to give me time to transcribe them as accurately as possible.

At the end of our meeting the Lama gave me some advice that has been of great importance to me; I have related those parts that contain indications and clarifications that may also prove useful to others.

2. Advice on the Great Seal

Homage to the Diamond Fairy!

THE Great Seal cannot be taught, but you, worthy, intelligent Nāropa, who in facing hard trials patiently bear suffering, thanks to your devotion to the teacher, take these [words] to heart.

Does space rest on anything? In the same way, the Great Seal has nothing on which to rest. Remain relaxed in the natural unaltered state. If bonds are loosened, without doubt one is free.

When one observes the centre of space, one ceases seeing [everything else]. In the same way, if one observes consciousness with consciousness, thought forms dissolve and supreme awakening ensues.

Fog banks dissolve in space without going elsewhere or remaining anywhere. In the same way, thought forms arise from consciousness, but when one views one's consciousness, the wave of mental images dissolves.

The true nature of space has neither colour nor form and is not conditioned either by white or black. In the same way, the essence of one's consciousness has neither colour nor form and is not conditioned either by virtue or vice.

The heart of the sun, clear and limpid, cannot be obscured by the darkness of a thousand ages. In the same way, the clear light that is the essence of one's consciousness cannot be obscured by the cycle of ages.

Space is defined as "empty" but space is ineffable. In the same way, one's consciousness is designated "clear light," yet, there is nothing in it that can be defined saying, "It is thus."

So, from the very beginning the true nature of consciousness is like space, and there is nothing that does not converge in it.

Stop any physical movement and remain quietly in the natural state. You have nothing to say; sounds are empty, like an echo. You have nothing to think about; contemplate what transcends [the mind].

Your body empty as a bamboo cane, your consciousness beyond thoughts like the centre of space, relax in this state without losing [awareness] or keeping [anything in mind].

Consciousness without reference points is the Great Seal. Getting used to this state, one obtains supreme awakening.

The vision of the Great Seal, that is clear light, cannot be achieved by clinging to the dogmatic explanations and scriptures of the various systems, instructions, ethical rules, [philosophical studies], perfections and the esoteric tradition. In fact, the vision of the clear light is obscured by dogmatism.

Dogmatic observance of precepts means not keeping the real commitment. Being without fixations is freedom from dogmatism. [Thought] is like a wave that naturally arises and subsides.

If you don't lose awareness of the authentic value, beyond fixed ideas and rigid conduct, [spiritual] commitment is kept like a light dispelling darkness.

When one is free of dogmatism by no longer clinging to a conclusion, one beholds [the true meaning of] all the teachings.

Advice on the Great Seal

Penetrating this truth frees one from the cage of *saṁsāra*. Contemplating this truth burns everything that causes obscuration and hindrance. [Whoever achieves this realization] is called "lamp of the teaching."

Fools, who do not prize this truth, end up letting themselves get dragged away by the stream of *saṁsāra*. Poor fools [who have to endure] this unbearable suffering! If they wish to bring it to an end they must follow an expert guide and let the spiritual energy flow down into their heart. Then their consciousness will be free.

Oh, [living according to] the law of *saṁsāra* is meaningless and causes suffering. Whatever is done [in this way] has no value. So consider what is valuable and meaningful.

The supreme view is to transcend subject and object. The supreme meditation is not being distracted. The supreme conduct is the absence of effort. Realization of the goal is to be without hope or fear.

The true nature of consciousness is clarity beyond images. The goal of the path of awakened beings is achieved without a path to travel. Supreme awakening is realized without having anything to practise.

Oh, consider carefully worldly existence. It is transitory; like an illusion and a dream, there is nothing real. So repent and forsake worldly action. Completely cut ties of affection for your retinue and your country. Meditate alone in a mountain hermitage or in the forest.

Remain in the state where there is nothing on which to meditate. If you obtain what cannot be obtained you will have obtained the Great Seal.

Branches and leaves grow from the trunk of a great tree; a sharp cut at its root and all the branches wither. In the same way, cutting the mind at its roots, the leaves of *saṁsāra* wither.

A lamp dispels darkness accumulated over a thousand ages. In the same way, the one clear light of one's consciousness dispels the darkness and obstacles of ignorance accumulated over the ages.

Oh, it is not by the intellect that one beholds what transcends it; it is not by action that one understands what transcends it.

If you wish to attain what transcends intellect and action, cut the mind at its root and leave awareness naked. Let the turbid water of thoughts clear itself. Leave phenomenal reality as it is, without affirming or denying.

Phenomenal existence without attachment or rejection is the Great Seal.

The universal base is unborn, so it is free of conditioning by psychological imprints. Remain in the unborn essence without pride or scheming. Allow phenomena to appear naturally and mental images to dissolve.

The supreme view is complete freedom from dogmatism. The supreme meditation is vast boundless depth. The supreme conduct is breaking limits. The supreme goal is the natural state without any more expectations.

At the start [the mind of] a beginner is like a waterfall. Then, it becomes like the river Ganges, flowing gently. Finally, it is like rivers flowing [into the sea, when] mother and child meet.

Someone with lesser capacity, unable to remain in the natural state, should leave awareness in its essential condition by controlling the breath. [Moreover] through various methods of fixing the gaze and concentrating thought one controls the mind until awareness abides in the natural state.

Relying on the seal of action, the knowledge of emptiness and bliss arises; when the energies of means and wisdom come together, let them descend slowly, then be held, pulled back, brought back to the source and spread throughout the bodies. If, in this moment, there is no longer desire the knowledge of emptiness and bliss arises.

[Whoever practises in this way] will live long, without white hair, and will wax like the moon; he or she will have a luminous mien and the strength of a lion, will quickly obtain the common powers and will remain absorbed in supreme awakening.

May this advice on the essence of the Great Seal remain in the heart of those destined [to receive it].[1]

---

1. The colophon reads thus: "This advice by Śrī Tilopa, the spontaneously realized [master], on the Great Seal was transmitted by the teacher himself on the banks of the Ganges to the realized scholar Nāropa, the *paṇḍita* from Kashmir, once he had faced twelve ascetic trials. The Tibetan translator Marpa Chökyi Lodrö received the twenty-eight diamond stanzas from the great Nāropa at North Pulahari, where after revising them, he made a definitive translation." Marpa was the teacher of the famous Tibetan mystic Milarepa.

3. Commentary

Homage to the Diamond Fairy!

Do you know who the "Diamond Fairy" (Vajraḍākinī) is? She is the feminine expression of the supreme divinity, of that which is unconditioned and unaltered and which constitutes the true way of being of all existence. Paying homage means recognizing her true nature. When Nāropa met Tilopa he needed greater and deeper knowledge of the feminine aspect of life. With the opening homage, the teacher also intends to point out this need and its meaning to him, which he resumes, in particular, at the end of the text.

> *The Great Seal cannot be taught, but you, worthy, intelligent Nāropa, who in facing hard trials patiently bear suffering, thanks to your devotion to the teacher, take these [words] to heart.*

In this tradition, the supreme divinity is referred to as the "Great Seal," because the sign of its presence marks every aspect of existence. And yet, paradoxically, nobody can show it or point to it directly precisely because it pervades and embraces all reality without being limited by anything and it transcends images, words and thoughts. Moreover, neither does the vision of the empty form (*stong gzugs*) of the feminine divinity, with which Nāropa wished to join in union, reveal the true indeterminable nature of the Great Seal.

Commentary

If you are not stupid, when I point my finger at a statue of Buddha you don't keep staring at my finger, nor do you come next to me to see the statue the way I see it; instead you follow my finger's direction and look at the statue, staying where you are. Nor do you think that it is the true state of Buddha. This is the way to regard and utilize the teachings on absolute reality left by the teachers.

Does space rest on anything? In the same way, the Great Seal has nothing on which to rest. Remain relaxed in the natural unaltered state. If bonds are loosened, without doubt one is free.

The most frequently recurrent symbol standing for the true nature of the divinity, that is absolute reality, is the sky. One can point at the moon in the sky, one can see it, but there is no way to determine empty space. If we want to measure space we need something within it to use as a reference point. Empty space, in which there is neither you nor anything else, does not rest on anything; it does not have any reference points. If that is the case, then how can one know the true divinity?

Tilopa says: "Remain relaxed in the natural unaltered state." Do not strive, do not try to adjust your body, your speech, your mind, or to change the place where you are. Just relax where you are, the way you are, natural.

What hinder us from recognizing the Great Seal of the true divinity are our bonds, our conditioning, and our personal limits; if we relax, they fall away naturally. Isn't this advice strange? All the religions teach that one has to fight against evil, to strive to improve, to repress the passions, to mortify the senses. Instead, Tilopa states that relaxing, without doing anything intentionally to modify reality, is enough. If you don't believe it, just try.

The moment something stirs up harmful thoughts or emotions is the time to test oneself by relaxing. Relaxing implies giving space, to yourself as well as to others. The problem dissolves in that space. If you stop giving importance to the problem it will certainly disappear. If it doesn't, it is because there is still tension.

> *When one observes the centre of space, one ceases seeing [everything else]. In the same way, if one observes consciousness with consciousness, thought forms dissolve and supreme awakening ensues.*

"When one observes the centre of space, one ceases seeing . . .," Tilopa tells his disciple, asking him to perform a very simple experiment. In fact, by focusing the attention on a point in empty space, one stops noticing the surrounding things. You only need try it to verify if it is so. Why don't you try now? Just one minute can be enough. . . .

This is just an example. Tilopa does not say it is necessary to train gazing at a point in space for as long as possible. Some people do, but that is not the case here. If you don't succeed in relaxing in the natural state by following his first instructions, then you must turn your attention within, on yourself; you don't need to look elsewhere. You just have to remain present to yourself.

You, who are thinking about the meaning of these words, are you aware of yourself at the same time? If you turn your attention within, then you can understand. Most people live in constant distraction, absorbed and conditioned by what they perceive, because they have no self-awareness, as if they were dreaming without realizing it.

When you regain awareness of yourself you feel being, you feel that you exist here and now, but you don't identify this pure feeling with what you perceive, thereby ending up forgetting yourself. Self-awareness is not distracted or disturbed by anything.

So, if you observe consciousness with consciousness, as just described, then thought forms, the mental fixations and disturbing fantasy images dissolve naturally, because they are no longer sustained by all of your personal attention.

Try right now! Close your eyes and think about something particularly pleasant. . . .

Now, notice that while you are thinking about that thing, you are, you exist. Don't you feel being?

If that thought is still present, let it go without forgetting yourself feeling being. . . .

In this way, sooner or later, all thoughts dissolve by themselves, because that is their nature.

Now try to repeat the experiment thinking about something unpleasant. . . .

That image too dissolves naturally, doesn't it? Every time this happens, awakening, liberation is achieved. It is like realizing that you are dreaming and no longer being conditioned by the unreal dream images. Once you free yourself of the illusion of all your dreams, in sleeping and in waking, you realize supreme enlightenment.

Fog banks dissolve in space without going elsewhere or remaining anywhere. In the same way, thought forms arise from consciousness, but when one views one's consciousness, the wave of mental images dissolves.

Fog arises in space, abides there and dissolves naturally. Mental images too, that veil the vision of true reality, have no other base than your own consciousness, in which they naturally resolve themselves.

Struggling with thoughts in order to eliminate them is like seeking to still water by stirring it; in this way, you only obtain the opposite result. Tilopa says it is enough to turn your attention on yourself, to remain present to yourself; when you view your consciousness as if you were observing the centre of space, the wave of mental images dissolves.

It is very important to verify this advice for yourself. To do this you must not get distracted, you must be aware, be present to yourself. This is the only way to understand the actual sense and practical value of Tilopa's words.

The true nature of space has neither colour nor form and is not conditioned either by white or black. In the same way, the essence of one's consciousness has neither colour nor form and is not conditioned either by virtue or vice.

Now, observe space: has it got a form or colour of its own? Do the light and dark clouds really change the true nature of space in which they appear and disappear?

Tilopa says that when you observe consciousness with consciousness, you discover it has neither colour nor form and is not conditioned either by virtue or vice, just like space.

One's true nature, one's real Self, is not the body, sensations, emotions, ideas or thoughts, with which one identifies the individual personality. So, if you perceive something when you observe consciousness, know that that is not your true impersonal essence. You must learn to stop identifying yourself with what you perceive and merely remain a pure witness to reality as it is. This is possible if you are present to yourself.

When you remain relaxed, being present to yourself, as if you were in space, then you understand that your true essence has nothing to do with the black clouds of vice or the white clouds of virtue that mark the personality. They are only mental images superimposed on true reality that, in itself, is free of all determinations. So, what need is there to struggle to improve yourself?

You think you've got vices and virtues. You try to get rid of the vices and to acquire the virtues. But vices and virtues are merely aspects of the personality, that is as changeable and transient as the clouds. Your divine essence is impersonal and by its very nature free of the chain of vices and virtues, like space that remains unaltered.

Commentary

> *The heart of the sun, clear and limpid, cannot be obscured by the darkness of a thousand ages. In the same way, the clear light that is the essence of one's consciousness cannot be obscured by the cycle of ages.*

According to ancient Indian cosmology, the manifestation of the universe follows cyclical laws. Buddhists give a generic definition of all the cycles, both the major and the minor ones, as "ages" (*kalpa*). The text refers to "the darkness of a thousand ages." This expression designates both periods in which life does not manifest and those in which life manifests but no totally awakened being, no Buddha, appears. During these dark phases, the heart of the sun does not undergo any change, it is both the energy centre emanating the visible sun and the essence or potentiality of awakening.

Your true nature is divine, pure from the beginning of any cycle, whether of the cosmos, of the planet, of your manifold existences or of this single existence; its light abides unaltered even through the succession of all the dark periods.

This allegory means that you should never despair, never let yourself get sad or dejected. You should face the dark moments of life bravely, trusting in the light that is always shining in your heart and in that of all beings. Pure faith is awareness of the divine essence that pervades all existence. This light is all you need to remember, venerate and contemplate. This light is all you need to call upon, with joy in your heart and certainty in your mind.

> *Space is defined as "empty" but space is ineffable. In the same way, one's consciousness is designated "clear light," yet, there is nothing in it that can be defined saying, "It is thus."*

The essence of your consciousness is divine, luminous, pure like empty space, but the word "empty" is not the true emptiness of space. In the same way, in terms of your true nature there is nothing in it that can be defined by saying, "It is thus."

The word "Buddha" is not the Buddha. The word "Christ" is not the Christ. The corresponding concepts too are not what they represent. The idea of God is not the true divinity. Whoever clings to sensations, thoughts, images or words can be compared to an idiot who mistakes his reflection in a mirror for a real person. This mistake frequently happens! This is the birthplace of intolerance in the name of truth. But take heed, because one can also become intolerant in the name of tolerance. What can you do to avoid this error or to overcome it? Remain like space, without fixing on the idea of emptiness or of the clarity of phenomena.

> *So, from the very beginning the true nature of consciousness is like space, and there is nothing that does not converge in it.*

In Buddhist philosophy, the original material element from which all phenomena issue, in which every concrete thing exists and resolves itself at the end of the cycle, is called "space." This fundamental element constitutes the symbol of the Great Seal, of absolute reality that is one's divine essence.

If the foregoing advice is not enough, if you are still asking yourself how to remain in your natural state as in space, then the words that follow could prove very useful, at least to someone determined to put them into practice:

> *Stop any physical movement and remain quietly in the natural state. You have nothing to say; sounds are empty, like an echo. You have nothing to think about; contemplate what transcends [the mind].*

You should know that in the natural state there is nothing to seek deliberately, no shadow of any striving, and there is nothing to correct in terms of the body, voice and mind. So, let your body relax in a comfortable posture: "Stop any physical movement and remain quietly," Tilopa says.

In general, meditation teachers advise at least to sit with the back straight, but Tilopa does not give even this instruction, because every individual has his or her own sensibility that must be respected in order not to create any psychophysical tension. If you listen to your body, you will be able to understand for yourself which is the best posture to take up at any given moment.

As regards the voice, Tilopa is equally peremptory: "You have nothing to say," neither prayers, nor *mantras*, chants nor anything else. In fact, sounds are empty, like an echo, because the true nature of reality is not the words that designate it.

Likewise, the same principle applies to the mind: "You have nothing to think about," Tilopa asserts, not about the divinity, nor the teacher, not about any symbol, concept or thing. In fact, the Great Seal transcends the mind.

> *Your body empty as a bamboo cane, your consciousness beyond thoughts like the centre of space, relax in this state without losing [awareness] or keeping [anything in mind].*

If you leave your body quietly in a comfortable position, at a certain point it will seem light, insubstantial, and empty as a bamboo cane.

If you stop creating thoughts deliberately and allow them to appear and disappear in a natural way, the feeling of your consciousness will remain firm, not disturbed by thoughts, like observing the centre of space, whereby one ceases seeing everything else.

Relaxing in this way in your natural state, take care not to lose awareness or keep anything in your mind. Leave everything as it is without falling into a state of torpor or letting yourself get distracted by thoughts. If you do get distracted, don't worry, because worry is a thought like the others, and, in any case, the moment you notice you have got distracted you are already present to yourself.

Try this right now!

If these words resound in your ears and echo in your mind, if they enhance your knowledge, if they fill your notebook and your mouth, unless they spur you to give all of this up, then they are not sacred words but worldly ones. Come on, close your notebook and stop looking at me! Silence. . . .

> *Consciousness without reference points is the Great Seal. Getting used to this state, one obtains supreme awakening.*

The Great Seal of true divinity is like boundless empty space; it reveals itself spontaneously in consciousness without reference points. When do we have reference points? When the mind clings to predetermined goals and hopes to accomplish them, to particular patterns and strives to adhere to them, to images of itself, of others, of things, and continues to cherish them.

The natural state of consciousness is free of the mind's illusions. Getting used to this natural state we learn to relax, letting thoughts dissolve spontaneously. In this way, attachment to one's own fixations loosens, bonds get unbound and, without doubt, one is free. But beware: the concept of what supreme awakening should be, too, is a reference point! Do you remember what Tilopa says right at the start? "The Great Seal cannot be taught." Whoever claims the opposite is profane, and if he is convinced of it, then he is deceiving himself as well as others.

> *The vision of the Great Seal, that is clear light, cannot be achieved by clinging to the dogmatic explanations and scriptures of the various systems, instructions (sūtra), ethical rules (vinaya), [philosophical studies (abhidharma)], perfections (pāramitā) and the esoteric tradition (tantra). In fact, the vision of the clear light is obscured by dogmatism.*

The clear light of the Great Seal cannot be obscured by the cycle of ages; nevertheless, one's understanding of its nature is hindered by dogmatism. Tilopa seems an iconoclast, but, really, he is proclaiming a hallowed principle; attachment to

Commentary

any common or esoteric system is a limitation because the truth transcends any barrier, it is not tied to any formulations, words, concepts, images or particular conduct, nor does it consist in any mystical experience. Whoever thinks one can achieve it by clinging to the dogmatic explanations and scriptures of any religion, doctrine or discipline will never accomplish it.

In our dimension, everything is transient and subject to the law of constant flux, so the various systems are too. Nevertheless, it is said that religion is like a ferry and the teacher is compared to a ferryman, both are necessary to reach the other shore. But what if there are no shores?

Tilopa doesn't use shores as an example. For him, ultimate reality is like boundless space, in terms of which the various systems are like clouds: some are lighter, some darker. He also says that awareness of the real truth is like the sun high in the sky, so bright that man cannot look straight at it without losing his sight; that is why there are clouds . . . and sunglasses. Tilopa invites us to be that awareness, to be the radiant sun in all-pervading boundless space.

As long as you conceive consciousness as something individual, a person or an "I" to analyse, satisfy, purify, punish, eliminate or deify, then you cannot be consciousness itself, in which there is no division between subject and object. Don't bother with shores, clouds and sunglasses and be like the sun in space.

> *Dogmatic observance of precepts means not keeping the real commitment. Being without fixations is freedom from dogmatism. [Thought] is like a wave that naturally arises and subsides.*

> *If you don't lose awareness of the authentic value, beyond fixed ideas and rigid conduct, [spiritual] commitment is kept like a light dispelling darkness.*

When one clings to a system in a dogmatic way, there are also precepts to observe. Obeying rules is like living in prison. In some cases, when someone is unable to live spontaneously in a considerate and respectful way, then it can be useful to have certain rules. However, they do not lead to freedom.

The true commitment (*samaya*) Tilopa speaks of consists in being free of conditioning by one's fixations, judgements and emotions. When you no longer cling to any image of yourself, of others and of any thing, then you behold consciousness free of dogmatism and you fly out of the prison of rigid precepts.

You do not need to strive to eliminate conditioning images. In fact, thoughts dissolve naturally like waves; if you stop stirring up water, that is, your psychic energy, with worrying, hopes and fears and striving to achieve your realization, then the waves come to rest by themselves.

The truth does not lie in rules. "Authentic value" lies only in consciousness, never outside it. When you are aware of this, you abandon fixed ideas and rigid conduct, but without relinquishing your spiritual commitment; it shines spontaneously, without any effort or tension, like a lamp that instantly dispels all darkness.

When one is free of dogmatism by no longer clinging to a conclusion, one beholds [the true meaning of] all the teachings.

The sundry teachings certainly have an authentic value but you cannot discover it as long as you remain tied to their words, concepts, images and norms. Their value lies in the universal truth that transcends the dogmas of different doctrines and the conclusions drawn by man's reasoning.

Penetrating this truth frees one from the cage of saṁsāra. *Contemplating this truth burns everything that causes obscuration and hindrance. [Whoever achieves this realization] is called "lamp of the teaching."*

Awareness of the universal truth is what frees you from the cage of *saṁsāra*, from the prison of conditioning. It is the

Commentary

clear light that shines in the consciousness of all human beings. Whoever beholds it no longer has any dark moments because one remains united to the source of all light. Such a being is the true "lamp of the teaching," Tilopa tells us.

> *Fools, who do not prize this truth, end up letting themselves get dragged away by the stream of* saṁsāra. *Poor fools [who have to endure] this unbearable suffering! If they wish to bring it to an end they must follow an expert guide and let the spiritual energy flow down into their heart. Then their consciousness will be free.*

Those who do not recognize the universal truth of inner freedom and let themselves get dragged away by the stream of *saṁsāra* in their continuous search for material and spiritual well-being, are fools. The wheel of fortune spins ceaselessly: prosperity and misery, fame and infamy, happiness and despair, beauty and ugliness, virtue and vice, birth and death, heaven and hell. Fools, who do not discern true freedom, cannot help but undergo all of this. If they wish to bring to an end the painful process of illusory becoming, then "they must follow an expert guide and let the spiritual energy flow down into their heart." What does Tilopa mean by these words?

He is explaining to his disciple, Nāropa, that there are persons, both lay and religious, who cannot accept the foregoing advice as true and valid because they are convinced they have to become other than what they are and that they can do this by striving to change the present in view of the final achievement.

It would be useful for those with such a worldly outlook to follow a teacher, recognizing him or her as the perfect realization of their own spiritual ideal and opening to the energy of the teacher's aura, imagining the light of his or her pure influence penetrating their heart until they feel at one with the teacher.

Just as contact with blazing coal turns a piece of metal incandescent, so contact with the teacher's limpid consciousness purifies one's mind, allowing the emergence of that state of pure awareness which alone enables one to understand the nature of the Great Seal.

This devotional meditation is called "identification with the teacher" (*guru-yoga*), it is connected with the first esoteric initiation and it comprises the essence of the "seal of commitment" (*samayamudrā*). Nāropa practised it intensively and for a long time, visualizing his teacher in the form of the divine couple called Cakrasaṁvara, in whom he contemplated the union of all the teachers and manifold divine manifestations.

I received the first initiation, the "vase empowerment" (*bum dbang*), at the age of seven from my main teacher, the abbot of the monastery I had entered the year before.

He did not confer the four initiations of the Higher Tantras (*anuttarayoga*) all together, as most of the Lamas do according to modern usage, but rather only gave the initiations he deemed necessary, and at different times, in accord with the ancient rule observed by the great teacher Padmasambhava. To me the teacher bestowed all the four.

From the moment I received the vase empowerment, I had to undertake the commitment to meditate daily on my identification with the teacher in the male form of the divine "Diamond Being" (Vajrasattva), at the same time imagining all the world as his paradise and all beings as his peaceful and wrathful manifestations. It was very important for me not to get distracted from the principle of identifying with my teacher after the meditation but to continue instead to deem everything as divine by nature, without discriminating between friend and foe, pleasant and unpleasant, higher and lower.

This practice is taught in many religions but, nowadays, very few people live out its true meaning all the time. Those who think they are able to should observe themselves during the day to see how free they are from the net of discrimination.

Commentary

> Oh, [living according to] the law of saṁsāra *is meaningless and causes suffering. Whatever is done [in this way] has no value. So consider what is valuable and meaningful.*

As long as you go on making discriminations you are still conditioned by desires and fears, liking and disliking, personal experiences and knowledge, in the unceasing quest for self-affirmation. Such a life is nothing but selfish, worldly action, devoid of any spiritual value. What then has meaning? What are the true values?

> *The supreme view is to transcend subject and object. The supreme meditation is not being distracted. The supreme conduct is the absence of effort. Realization of the goal is to be without hope or fear.*

Someone with a spiritual point of view will probably answer that true values are religious ones. But in what does religion consist? If we consider religion from the viewpoint of *saṁsāra*, then one could believe in a personal God, in an individual soul, in a realized teacher, in a perfect abstract or ideal reality to contemplate or to accomplish for one's own benefit. All these conceptions are characterized by the separation between subject and object, I and others, oneself and what one hopes to achieve. "The supreme view," Tilopa says, "is to transcend subject and object."

If we are distracted while we are praying, reciting *mantras*, visualizing symbols and sacred images, performing rituals, controlling the breath or whatever then we are not really meditating. Many meditation instructors teach mental concentration as a way not to get distracted, nevertheless there is a subtle kind of distraction that consists precisely in focusing one's attention on a concrete or imaginary object. "The supreme meditation is not being distracted," says Tilopa.

If we strive to comply with precepts, we do not live by them spontaneously. When our conduct is not a natural expression of the impersonal divine essence but instead is conditioned by ambition and prejudice this always implies striving, tension, contrast, struggle, imposition. Tilopa says, "supreme conduct is absence of effort."

If we cherish expectations and fears regarding spiritual realization, then we need to understand that the true goal is already present here and now, because it is nothing other than our own original nature. This awareness is the lamp of pure faith, luminous consciousness of the eternal present that instantly dispels the dark illusion of the past and of the future. "Realization of the goal is to be without hope or fear," says Tilopa.

Why does Tilopa say this, immediately after telling us it is possible to accomplish liberation by following a teacher and letting his or her spiritual energy flow down into one's heart? Isn't this a contradiction?

Nāropa was very intelligent and deeply devoted to his teacher, but he was also very headstrong. For eight years he had been abbot of Nālandā, an important Buddhist monastery in India. At that time, he was very knowledgeable about the scriptures, both common and esoteric, about logic, the philosophies of the different schools and the meditation techniques and rituals of the Buddhist religion and furthermore he had already written his learned works. Nevertheless, one fine day, while he was meditating on the sacred scriptures he understood that, actually, he had not yet realized their real meaning. So he abandoned all his books and duties at the monastery and set off in search of his real teacher. This text is a collection of the first counsels on the Great Seal that he received from Tilopa on the banks of the Ganges.

Being very skilful in dialectics and a zealous defender of Buddhist orthodoxy in debates with the Hindus, Nāropa was obstinate and stubborn in upholding his own convictions; his teacher was well aware of this and that was why he patiently, but firmly, started work on demolishing his disciple's dogmatic position.

Commentary

In these last counsels, Tilopa utilizes paradox and contradiction expressly to point out to Nāropa the limits of his mind. Identification with the teacher or, in any case, with a being deemed to be divine, implies a separation between subject and object, otherwise there would be no other with which to identify yourself; it implies distraction from your true nature, otherwise you would not feel the need to identify yourself with another; it implies effort, otherwise you would not strive to practise meditation; it implies hope and fear, otherwise you would stay the way you are.

> *The true nature of consciousness is clarity beyond images. The goal of the path of awakened beings is achieved without a path to travel. Supreme awakening is realized without having anything to practise.*

Tilopa had understood that in the natural state of consciousness the senses function fully but that the perception of phenomena is no longer filtered by mental images. In fact, the mind's images are subjective and misleading projections on reality as it is. If this is the true nature of things, then why do you need to imagine your teacher or a symbol of him or her?

The spiritual path too is a mental image, and travelling the path implies effort. It is only by giving up the concept of a path and the striving to travel along it that you reach the goal of the true path on which there is no journey. Why the need, then, to identify yourself with your teacher?

Finally, according to Tilopa, in order to realize supreme awakening there is no need to develop any particular powers through any specific ascetic, mystical, magical or other types of practices. Why the need, then, to train yourself to meditate on your teacher's spiritual energy by identifying with his or her state of consciousness?

Because Nāropa was stubborn, he did not understand. So Tilopa offered him another clue:

Oh, consider carefully worldly existence. It is transitory; like an illusion and a dream, there is nothing real. So repent and forsake worldly action. Completely cut ties of affection for your retinue and your country. Meditate alone in a mountain hermitage or in the forest.

Nāropa was pleased to hear that, at last, his teacher was giving him precise instructions on the method to use and thought that on retreat he could put his advice into practice, mainly by identifying himself with his teacher's state of consciousness during his meditation. But Tilopa continued:

Remain in the state where there is nothing on which to meditate. If you obtain what cannot be obtained you will have obtained the Great Seal.

Unfortunately, Nāropa's armour was so thick that Tilopa's words could not reach his heart. In fact, on account of the way he had interpreted the previous instructions on the sky he thought they meant that once he had identified himself with his teacher he should focus his mind on empty space.

Nāropa knew that identifying oneself with one's teacher by meditating on his or her symbolic image, whether human or divine, is the essence of the "creation process,"[1] the first phase of the esoteric meditation method, and that focusing on empty space is the basis of the "completion process,"[2] the second and final phase.

He believed that Tilopa's preceding instructions were mainly concerned with the second process, when one meditates without anything on which to meditate, precisely because it involves concentration on the sky devoid of clouds, giving rise, sooner or later, to a vision of the empty form of the divinity, that he called *mahāmudrā*.

Branches and leaves grow from the trunk of a great tree; a sharp

---

1. Tib. *bskyed rim*; Skt. *utpattikrama*.
2. Tib. *rdzogs rim*; Skt. *utpannakrama*.

> *cut at its root and all the branches wither. In the same way, cutting the mind at its roots, the leaves of* saṁsāra *wither.*

Because of his conditioning by the knowledge he had gathered Nāropa continued in his misinterpretation, so Tilopa tried to enable him to understand that all experiences and convictions are like branches and leaves of the tree of *saṁsāra*; the mind is their underlying base, which needs to be cut sharply at a stroke.

Nāropa was convinced that in order to dispel the darkness he had accumulated over many lifetimes in unending ages, due to his ignorance of the true nature of things, he had to accumulate good deeds and wisdom over the course of countless lives. That was why he did not grasp the true meaning of the previous example. So Tilopa reiterated the same principle using the example of the single lamp that dispels the darkness of ages.

> *A lamp dispels darkness accumulated over a thousand ages. In the same way, the one clear light of one's consciousness dispels the darkness and obstacles of ignorance accumulated over the ages.*

In general, in terms of the ages the lamp represents a Buddha, whose coming brings spiritual light, and this was how Nāropa immediately interpreted the example. However, Tilopa explained that the true lamp is awareness of one's own divine essence that instantaneously dispels the darkness of ignorance and the obstacles of the ensuing negative actions accumulated in the past, even during infinite previous existences.

> *Oh, it is not by the intellect that one beholds what transcends it; it is not by action that one understands what transcends it.*

You too, like Nāropa the disciple, are seeking the truth with your intellect, conditioned by the knowledge that you have accumulated; you too are striving to do something to accomplish your life's aim.

> *If you wish to attain what transcends intellect and action, cut the mind at its root and leave awareness naked. Let the turbid water of*

> *thoughts clear itself. Leave phenomenal reality as it is, without affirming or denying.*

If you are still asking yourself how to transcend the intellect and action, listen to Tilopa: "cut the mind at its root and leave awareness naked." Here is the essence of his advice on the Great Seal.

Cutting the mind at its root means breaking the chain of conditioning, sharply cutting your disordered habits, your negative thoughts and harmful emotions. You can't manage this by striving to correct your conduct but only by remaining aware in a state of pure observation, no longer impulsively reacting to stimuli.

Now, let's try an experiment. I'll put some earth into this glass of clean water. As you can see the water gets turbid, even though its nature is limpid.

If we leave the glass still for a while the water clears itself. . . .

If we shake the glass, the water gets turbid again. . . .

The glass is like our psychophysical organism and our psychic energy is like the water. Our emotions, negative thoughts and dogmatic ideas are like the earth that sullies the water. There is no way for the water to get clear by stirring it or shaking the glass. That is why Tilopa's essential advice consists in only one counsel: "Leave phenomenal reality as it is, without affirming or denying."

Don't cling to sensations and thoughts; do not repress them by inhibiting yourself. Just be aware, notice what is moving inside you and observe your impulses and reaction mechanisms without changing anything or getting distracted.

> *Phenomenal existence without attachment or rejection is the Great Seal.*

If you put this advice into practice immediately, in a radical way, without forgoing the experiences you think you need or getting caught up in them, you can really understand what

Tilopa means when he asserts that existence is the Great Seal. You should know that every aspect of life, any being or thing, is a manifestation of the supreme divinity. Everything is a sign of the transcendent!

I am no more the teacher of the Great Seal than is the leper you meet in the road, the poor child playing in the middle of rubbish, the beggar to whom you give alms, the mangy dog you chase away, the emotions that arouse you, the dreams that delude you, the fears that pursue you, the hopes that entice you, the pleasures that seduce you and all the rest. If you stopped discriminating and heeded the signs, you would understand.

> *The universal base is unborn, so it is free of conditioning by psychological imprints. Remain in the unborn essence without pride or scheming. Allow phenomena to appear naturally and mental images to dissolve.*

The Great Seal of the true divinity is the universal ground, the base of everything that exists, comparable to the original space of Buddhist cosmology. Being absolute and primordial reality, the supreme base is not preceded by a cause, so it is not born from something else pre-existing. Not being subject to saṁsāra, it is not conditioned by anything, not even by those traces which, impressed on the mind by experiences, determine behaviour. So, do not seek the Great Seal with the mind or in experiences, however sublime they might seem. Just remain in the natural state, in the boundless space of your causeless essence.

If, by chance, you should have some extraordinary, mystical, powerful, revelatory, luminous experience and you think it has brought you nearer to supreme reality, you should know that your small ego is inflating with pride, even though you haven't noticed it yet.

If you believe your nearness to the divine, the unborn, the absolute, can be measured by the amount of good deeds you have done and the wisdom you have accumulated, and you want to know what level of evolution you have attained you should know that your egocentric mind is about to trap you in its closely-woven net.

If you want to save yourself from the fiendish trap laid by the proud, calculating mind, mark Tilopa's words: "Allow phenomena to appear naturally and mental images to dissolve." You already know what this advice means, now it is up to you to put it into practice in your daily life. If you still have doubts about how to live the teaching of the Great Seal, ponder the following four aphorisms carefully:

The supreme view is complete freedom from dogmatism. The supreme meditation is vast boundless depth. The supreme conduct is breaking limits. The supreme goal is the natural state without any more expectations.

1. Go ahead and study any viewpoint in the world if you feel the need to, but do not turn any of them into an absolute because a fixed, rigid thought system is always limited. The truth of the Great Seal lies in freedom from the chains of convictions, but even asserting this can become a chain if it is used as a slogan or seized as a banner.

2. Go ahead and try various meditation techniques if it helps you in your growth, but do not stop at their limited experiences because the Great Seal has no support, no means and no end. The final meditation is not fixing on any meditative experience, but if you grasp non-meditation too you have set up a new barrier.

3. Go ahead and espouse rules if you think they can be useful, but don't get trapped by them because every aspect of life is marked with the sign of the Great Seal. True purity consists in your inner attitude, but don't break the law, respect others' customs and feel free to embrace them, if circumstances demand it and it doesn't harm anybody.

4. Go ahead and pursue your goals if they seem noble and just, but remember that psychological tension is a disease.

If you meet with success don't swell with pride, if you don't, or if you lose it, don't lose heart. The true goal is to transcend your ego's ambition, but if you expect others to live like you, then you haven't yet understood that everybody has to play their part in the great orchestra of impersonal life.

At the start [the mind of] a beginner is like a waterfall. Then, it becomes like the river Ganges, flowing gently. Finally, it is like rivers flowing [into the sea, when] mother and child meet.

Whoever puts Tilopa's advice into practice can discover that, at the start, one's mind is like a waterfall of thoughts and images; there is no need to try to stop it by blocking its flow because there is nothing in it to worry about. It is like having taken the lid off the boiling pot of the mind.

If you lower the flame by relaxing ever more deeply and completely, you can discover that, slowly, your mind becomes like a great river flowing gently. Thoughts, fantasies, memories and dreams continue to arise but not impetuously, so that you are able to sail freely on the water, and even to swim in it, staying aware both in outer quiet and tumult and in inner tranquillity and movement.

These experiences are common enough but only some contemplatives and mystics undergo those that follow, while most human beings only have them at the moment of death or afterwards.

When the flame under the pot becomes so low that the water stops boiling, self-awareness freely abides in a state of emptiness of the mind that can be compared to the space between two thoughts. In this state of consciousness, thoughts can arise when needed, but when they are no longer needed they dissolve spontaneously into emptiness. During the whole process one's awareness abides undisturbed.

Then, when the flame burning under the pot is put out and the well-cooked contents end up in the stomachs of one or more people for their nourishment, this is the moment when subject and object become one single thing. In this case, we say that the river flows into the sea. Your imagination's fancies dissolve, your mind loses any sense of separation from everything else and the individual consciousness returns to the universal consciousness like a child finding its mother again.

> *Someone with lesser capacity, unable to remain in the natural state, should leave awareness in its essential condition by controlling the breath. [Moreover] through various methods of fixing the gaze and concentrating thought one controls the mind until awareness abides in the natural state.*

According to Tilopa, there are people able to put the essential advice on the Great Seal into practice without having to meditate on a teacher or on the transience and illusoriness of existence and who do not need to cut their emotional ties and go into solitary retreat in order to relax and rediscover their spiritual essence. These people are endowed with higher capacity than others.

There are also many people who, in Tilopa's words, being unable to remain in the natural state through the foregoing instructions do not belong to the higher or average categories but, instead, to the lower one and so need still more methods.

It should be clear that this classification of people into categories is purely methodological and pragmatic, inasmuch as it regards only different cognitive procedures and does not imply any value judgements about the spiritual level of single individuals. It is like saying that there are people who are more intuitive and others who are more rational or more emotional; the more intuitive are superior, only because they can understand before others the true meaning of the essence that transcends rational thought and the emotions.

Those belonging to the third category can train in gradually gaining control over their breath, regulating its phases and increasing the apnoea because, to quote an ancient

Commentary

Indian dictum, the breath is like a horse and the mind is its rider.

Another gradual practice consists in directing the gaze downwards, straight ahead or upwards, while concentrating the mind on a concrete or visualized object or on empty space, or outside oneself or within the body.

The main aim of these techniques is to manage to remain in the state of pure awareness with the mind empty or with thoughts and sensations present but not giving rise to distraction. Some of these methods are also utilized in the esoteric tradition in relation to the second initiation and to the "seal of the teaching" (*dharmamudrā*).

I received the second initiation, the "secret empowerment" (*gsang dbang*), at the age of ten. Scrupulously following my teacher's explanations on the breathing methods, the physical postures and the visualizations, first of all I learnt to concentrate my psychic energy in the energy centres (*cakra*) in the head, throat, heart and navel and, subsequently, to bring it up from the sexual centre to the centre in the head.

It is very important to adopt methods of proven validity. Ideally, one should follow instructions from a teacher of the discipline in order to avoid damaging one's physical health and mental equilibrium through harmful or badly executed breathing and concentration exercises.

> *Relying on the seal of action, the knowledge of emptiness and bliss arises; when the energies of means and wisdom come together, let them descend slowly, then be held, pulled back, brought back to the source and spread throughout the bodies. If, in this moment, there is no longer desire the knowledge of emptiness and bliss arises.*

The third esoteric initiation enables you to practise the "seal of action" (*karmamudrā*), that is, heterosexual intercourse, accepted by tāntric Buddhism as a possible means of deliverance, contrary to the common tradition founded exclusively on monastic institutions.

When Nāropa received these last counsels he already knew about the path of sexual union consecrated through esoteric ritual but he was still attached to women and, moreover, he was convinced that full spiritual awakening was not possible without the experience of sexual pleasure, suitably controlled and channelled upwards.

He had yet to understand that nobody advances spiritually by means of sexual pleasure. However, sex can enable one to overcome great obstacles if it is the expression of true love. Love is sublime when, rather than setting subject and object in a dualistic relationship based on domination, exploitation and possessiveness, it is instead a feeling that harmonizes them in a non-dual relationship of equality, fusion and boundlessness.

To this end, esoteric Buddhism considers sexual intercourse as the union of the complementary aspects of the divinity, male means (*upāya*) and female wisdom (*prajñā*). During intercourse, the man and woman visualize themselves as divine beings. The image of the Diamond Fairy is one of the many feminine representations of the divinity. Moreover, according to the Tantras one must learn not to dissipate sexual energy but instead retain it and lead it back from the sexual organ to the head.

When in love play there is both freedom and understanding of its sacredness, at a certain point passionate desire dissolves like a cloud in the sky, yet the feeling of bliss continues to vibrate. Tilopa says that, in this moment, the non-dual knowledge of emptiness and bliss arises, that is the state of pure awareness.

> [Whoever practises in this way] will live long, without white hair, and will wax like the moon; he or she will have a luminous mien and the strength of a lion, will quickly obtain the common powers and will remain absorbed in supreme awakening.

Commentary

Tilopa asserts that to consummate sexual relations, bearing in mind the preceding guidance, cannot lead to physical deterioration or psychic derangement.

When I received the third tāntric initiation, I was a monk of twelve, nevertheless, my teacher authorized me both to imagine sexual intercourse and to experience it in reality congruent with the precepts of the initiation. My tradition does not find any contradiction in this, because monastic vows are external and, thus, are not broken by the observance of tāntric commitment, that is secret.

The basic difference between a tāntric monk or nun and a lay person is that the former does not set up a family. In any case, a genuine practitioner of the orthodox Tantras is not a libertine, he or she maintains chastity but without being bound by the rigid rules of monastic ethics. True chastity consists in perfect control of one's mind, one's psychic energy. For a long time now, the monasteries have been full of dissolute people while outside their cramped boundaries there are many lay people who live chastely even without ever having taken vows.

May this advice on the essence of the Great Seal remain in the heart of those destined [to receive it].

On receiving this advice, Nāropa devoted several years to practising the meditations connected with the esoteric initiations mentioned above. He pursued his own gradual path with devotion and determination, until, one fine day, he intuited the real meaning of Tilopa's teachings on the essence of consciousness that transcends intellect and action. At this point, Nāropa received the final advice on the fourth initiation and, at last, embarked on the short path of instantaneous understanding.

4. The Treasury of Hymns

Homage to glorious Diamond Being!
Homage to the Great Seal, immutable self-awareness!

ALL the factors of existence spring from the substance of the Great Seal and dissolve into it. It is not something, nor is it nothing, because it is beyond any determination. As it cannot be known by the mind, do not seek the meaning.

All phenomena are by their very nature false so there is no beginning and no end.

Here, whatever the mind can know is not considered as the true way of being of reality; true reality is not [made known] by the teacher nor is it [known] by the disciple.

Do not conceive of this state either as conscious or as unconscious; understand instead that it is the one devoid of multiplicity. But if you cling to the one, just that will bind you.

I, Tilo, have nothing to teach. I do not stay secluded, neither am I without seclusion. My eyes are not open, nor are they shut. My consciousness is not altered, nor is it unamended.

Realize that the natural state cannot be known with the mind. If you understand that adventitious experiences, memories and knowledge are something false as regards true indeterminable reality, leave all these phenomena as they are. There is no misery or prosperity, no obtainment or loss.

Do not remain in the forest, practising asceticism. Bliss cannot be found by means of washing and ritual purity. Nor will worshipping deities gain you liberation. Understand the relaxation in which one does not grasp or reject anything.

The goal is awareness of one's true nature. The instant one achieves this understanding there is no longer any path to follow. Ordinary people who do not understand seek the goal elsewhere. Bliss is transcending hope and fear.

When the I-thought dissolves, dualistic vision ceases.

Without thinking, imagining, examining, judging, meditating, acting, hoping or fearing, the impulses of the intellect fixing on these [activities] spontaneously dissolve. It is thus that one achieves the primordial state.[1]

---

1. This is the colophon: "*The Treasury of Hymns*, composed by Tilopa, is complete. Independently translated [into Tibetan] by the Indian teacher Vairocana."

5. Commentary

Homage to glorious Diamond Being!
Homage to the Great Seal, immutable self-awareness!

DIAMOND being is a male divinity. Tilopa devoted the first homage of his final counsels to him because he saw that his disciple Nāropa was able to recognize the primordial completeness of his essence without needing to seek it in a female image.

The single diamond substance of all beings, one's real Self in which the male and female principles are inseparable, is pure awareness; it knows itself spontaneously because it is self-resplendent and it does not change over time because it is immutable.

All the factors of existence spring from the substance of the Great Seal and dissolve into it. It is not something, nor is it nothing, because it is beyond any determination. As it cannot be known by the mind, do not seek the meaning.

The Great Seal is not only the true nature of living beings but also the supreme substance of all reality. Just as there exists a primordial etheric element, there is also a metaphysical principle that constitutes the divine essence of beings and worlds, the total base of every thing. Nevertheless, the true divinity cannot be identified with a

Commentary

form, a name or a concept; neither can its existence be refuted on this account.

If an original, causeless principle did not exist, there would be no way to transcend the limits of apparent reality that is subject to becoming, however who can say in what it consists? Any personal effort aimed at realizing absolute reality is futile because it cannot be caught in the net of the human mind. Can the sky be grasped or circumscribed?

All phenomena are by their very nature false so there is no beginning and no end.

Imagine you are dreaming about a man who is trying to kill you; as it is a dream, he cannot really hurt you, so you don't have to defend yourself.

Don't think you have to renounce many ordinary life experiences because you believe they are incompatible with spiritual evolution. Nor should you think that, in actual fact, evil objectively exists independently of people's bad thoughts.

Someone might argue that, in any case, sooner or later you stop dreaming and that likewise, when a human being accomplishes total realization, for him or her life is definitively extinguished, because spiritual perfection is incompatible with existence. If you believe this line of reasoning is valid, then listen and reflect. Isn't it possible to dream with awareness? And does the end of a dream ever lead to death?

Now, look at this mirror. What image do you see? You know very well that it is only an image of your face, nevertheless the image goes on appearing. The obtuse might believe that the reflection is something real. In the same way, even the most intelligent people do not recognize the illusory nature of phenomena. Though there is someone who recognizes it, phenomena go on appearing. Do you understand the real reason why? All of reality, just as it appears, is nothing but the manifestation of the great mirror of the true divinity.

> *Here, whatever the mind can know is not considered as the true way of being of reality; true reality is not [made known] by the teacher nor is it [known] by the disciple.*

In the state of the Great Seal, anything the mind can know is not deemed the true way of being of reality. The reflection is not the mirror. Appearance is not true reality. How then can a teacher possibly transmit the supreme truth? If the teacher cannot enable you to know it, why go on relying on him or her? Is it up to the disciple to grasp it for him or herself? But how will he or she manage, since it is indeterminable like the sky?

> *Do not conceive of this state either as conscious or as unconscious; understand instead that it is the one devoid of multiplicity. But if you cling to the one, just that will bind you.*

If you assert that the state of the Great Seal is conscious, this means it is knowable and thus determinable. If you assert that it is unconscious, you deny its existence, as if it were a hare's horn that cannot be perceived because it does not really exist.

According to Tilopa, it is the one devoid of multiplicity because in that state of being one does not feel any separation between self and other, between this and that. But be careful: if you cling to the one, just that will bind you. The one the teacher is talking about is like the mirror; the one you can cling to with your mind is merely an image, like the reflection in a mirror.

Even the subtlest and deepest conviction is a trap. Any dogmatic position is like a cloud, covering the sky and obscuring the sun; do you think you can dissolve it or remove it by blowing at it? Or do you think you can sit on it in order to contemplate what is beyond it?

> *I, Tilo, have nothing to teach. I do not stay secluded, neither am I without seclusion. My eyes are not open, nor are they shut. My consciousness is not altered, nor is it unamended.*

Commentary

This is why Tilopa declares that he has nothing to teach; in him every kind of mental fixation has dissolved. Those who really understand the Great Seal can live in the midst of people without being perturbed, can keep their eyes wide open without seeing anything, and their consciousness, amended of mental delusions, cannot be altered by anything.

> *Realize that the natural state cannot be known with the mind. If you understand that adventitious experiences, memories and knowledge are something false as regards true indeterminable reality, leave all these phenomena as they are. There is no misery or prosperity, no obtainment or loss.*

The mind is like a reflection or a cloud. In itself, consciousness is like the clear, limpid mirror or the sun in the sky. Reflections and clouds are multiple phenomena, yet they manifest spontaneously in the one mirror or in the one sky. For this reason, Tilopa asserts that there is nothing to obtain or lose.

Why then do you go on refusing to live your life to the full, obstinately remaining isolated in the narrow refuge of your little ego? Tilopa urged his disciple thus, once he was ready to understand:

> *Do not remain in the forest, practising asceticism. Bliss cannot be found by means of washing and ritual purity. Nor will worshipping deities gain you liberation. Understand the relaxation in which one does not grasp or reject anything.*

Neither ablution, a rigid diet, ritual changing of clothes, sexual abstinence or any other kind of outward observance can guarantee the bliss of true inner purity. Nor will worshipping the various deities, that vary according to different religions, family traditions and individual preferences, gain you total liberation from the net of the mind that seeks its own deliverance.

There is only one thing you can do that won't feed the illusion of your small ego: understand the relaxation in which there is no grasping or rejecting anything. Take care, this is not a technique that your ego can use for its own growth, nor is it an instigation to licentiousness.

The true meaning of the relaxation Tilopa is talking about is only truly realized when you let go of the tight grip of your ego. If you relax in this way, the tension of attachment and aversion dissolves and the limpid nature of your consciousness shines like a mirror that reflects all things equally, without striving to hold onto some reflections and to eliminate others.

> *The goal is awareness of one's true nature. The instant one achieves this understanding there is no longer any path to follow. Ordinary people who do not understand seek the goal elsewhere. Bliss is transcending hope and fear.*

Awareness of one's true nature, the single divine essence present in every being, is the self-awareness of the opening homage. According to Tilopa, it is the only true goal of human life. On attaining it, one understands that, paradoxically, the point of arrival is the same as the point of departure. Every instant is departure and arrival at the same time. So, what sense is there in living awaiting some future realization?

Cease projecting yourself into future time, because this stops you from fully living the sacredness of the present. As long as you seek the goal in the future and outside yourself, you will never find peace. Listen to Tilopa: "Bliss is transcending hope and fear." The kingdom of Buddha, or of God, is already present, here and now, for those with the single eye of pure faith.

> *When the I-thought dissolves, dualistic vision ceases.*

A solid thing can collide with another solid thing. As long as you believe you are this or that, then conflict with something else is always possible. Be like the sky that embraces and pervades everything and you will see that the illusion of dualism will cease along with every kind of strife.

Commentary

> *Without thinking, imagining, examining, judging, meditating, acting, hoping or fearing, the impulses of the intellect fixing on these [activities] spontaneously dissolve. It is thus that one achieves the primordial state.*

There is nothing to do deliberately in order to be like space. Just let your mental fixations dissolve spontaneously like waves, "without thinking, imagining, examining, judging, meditating, acting, hoping or fearing," says Tilopa. The moment this takes place you achieve the primordial state, your true original and natural way of being.

If you go on thinking that this realization is an event in the future, you haven't yet understood the meaning of the Great Seal. If you are determined to understand it, then observe yourself within and be aware of when the wave of thought or of emotion surges in your mind; do not try either to sustain it or to restrain it, instead relax and let it dissolve naturally. If you succeed, don't grow proud because other, far higher waves could surge up. If you don't succeed, don't worry because the water is the same in the wave as in the calm depths. Now, go and be happy. . . .

GIUSEPPE BAROETTO (GB): Before leaving, I would like to ask you some questions.

LHÜNDRUP TENZIN (LT): Then, stay and ask your questions.

GB: If *Mahāmudrā* cannot be taught and the pure essence of consciousness cannot be pointed out, saying, "It is thus," why are we taught to recognize our true nature by turning our attention within?

LT: This is done in order to awaken from distraction by rediscovering full self-awareness in the state of self-liberation. Distraction means letting oneself be conditioned by dualistic thoughts, by all those thoughts that limit us, bind us, stop us flying freely in the sky like a great eagle.

GB: Keeping present to oneself doesn't seem a natural state to me because it needs effort.

LT: The effort is needed because the presence you are seeking to maintain is still dualistic. Overcome the separation between subject and object.

GB: But the non-dual presence you are talking about is a state of contemplation that does not easily occur at any moment.

LT: During contemplation you learn to merge your awareness with the great void, pure being that is the universal base, without reasoning, judging or visualizing anything. But, in daily life, you have to be able to integrate contemplation and action. You can't integrate because you think you have to realize a stable state of contemplation, and when you don't succeed you strive to avoid getting distracted by trying to remain present to yourself. But all of this is unnatural and implies a twofold inner division.

Don't get your mind stuck on the sense of presence. Otherwise, you will end up living in a state of consciousness where feeling yourself and feeling the other are separate. Your awareness remains split into a part that is turned towards the subject and another that looks at the object.

During daily life, turn your attention to yourself every now and again, when you notice you have let yourself get distracted by limiting thoughts, then integrate presence with your sundry activities. Freely merge feeling yourself with the act of seeing, hearing, smelling, tasting, thinking and experiencing emotions. When you integrate in this way you don't feel yourself as something separate, but you are simply yourself in the present moment.

Don't think that non-dual awareness is a particular state of consciousness that only contemplatives can reach; it is the state of being that anyone can experience when really being oneself in the present moment.

Mahāmudrā means being present without separating what you are from what you would like to be. When, instead of being yourself you are trying to be, you alter your natural state and live divided within, tormented between hope and fear so that you are not fully present. Don't seek what is already here. The true spiritual quest lies in not seeking.

GB: Yet, Tilopa seems to have realized a state of non-dual consciousness free of the illusion of the ego. Knowing that, inevitably meditation is practised with the aim of achieving that final realization.

LT: This is the mistake that is stopping you from being present here and now. If you were, you would understand that your ordinary consciousness itself is the goal. Absolute reality, that your venerable teacher calls *Dzogchen*, is omnipresent, so every aspect of life bears its indelible seal.

The mind perceives only one present, not everything. So, don't limit the present. Open your eyes and see: you are already a Buddha! The problem lies in your mind that thinks it is not yet what it wishes to become.

Tilopa understood the true meaning of the Great Seal when he experienced the diamond contemplation, in which consciousness is unceasingly awake but free of mental images. Yet, he transmitted the teaching of the Great Seal to Nāropa from their very first meeting because he knew that the truth of one's original essence is always valid.

You, too, could understand the truth of the Great Seal, right now, if you could only stop judging yourself; consider every aspect of yourself with equanimity without refusing any part of yourself and, at last, let yourself be the divinity that you have always been.

GB: But, the moment I realize a thought is limiting me I have made a judgement.

LT: Don't bind your attention to that limiting thought to follow it by justifying it or to evade it by condemning it. Instead, be present to yourself with equanimity and relax, letting the thought dissolve by itself, naturally.

Dualistic thoughts are guides that can teach you something important because they too are expressions of the energy of the Great Seal. In order to contemplate the divinity in all beings, you must start with yourself; learn to be aware of yourself without judging yourself so that you will be able to understand others in the same way.

GB: For me, this contemplation of the divinity is only an idea that does not correspond with reality.

LT: An idea can be reality, if you are convinced of this. But you are not convinced of this because you think you are by nature limited, so you judge others in the same way. The difficulty I have with you, is similar to that Tilopa had with Nāropa. Listen with your heart to the words of someone who has understood, they are diamond words because they point out your true original nature, that is pure, limpid and perennial.

Time, the way you live it, is an illusion. From the very beginning you have had what you hope to obtain at the end of the wheel. "Buddha" is one who realizes this understanding. The divine Lord of the "Wheel of Time" (Kālacakra), free from birth and death, has always been seated on the central throne of your eternal heart. That is your diamond essence so you are already Diamond Being.

Call it God, if you prefer, or Allah, Great Spirit, Tao, Brahmā, Śiva, Viṣṇu, Cosmic Christ, Primordial Buddha or any other way and, if you don't want to give it a name, remain silent; but you should know that the ultimate sense does not change because the real original base is one and universal, transcendent yet immanent, ineffable yet luminous, omnipotent, all-embracing and omnipresent. The panacea, the remedy that cures all ills, is just this single awareness.

GB: If this is the truth, then why do I go on experiencing limitations, suffering and illusion?

LT: Buddha Śākyamuni, too, experienced them in the same way as you, otherwise he would not have been able to transcend them and then to point out the way of liberation. Without sleep, there is no awakening. Without *saṁsāra* or transmigration, there is no *nirvāṇa* or liberation. But you only awaken to your own Buddha-nature by learning not to separate *saṁsāra* and *nirvāṇa*.

You know that one of the many names given to the Primordial Buddha is Universal Goodness (Samantabhadra), precisely because it is present in all beings without any discrimination. Individual Buddhas manifest in the three moments of time by recognizing that single original base. So love yourself and all beings just as the Primordial Buddha, that is in every being, loves itself and all of life, so, you will understand the true sense of awakening to the state that is already awake. . . .

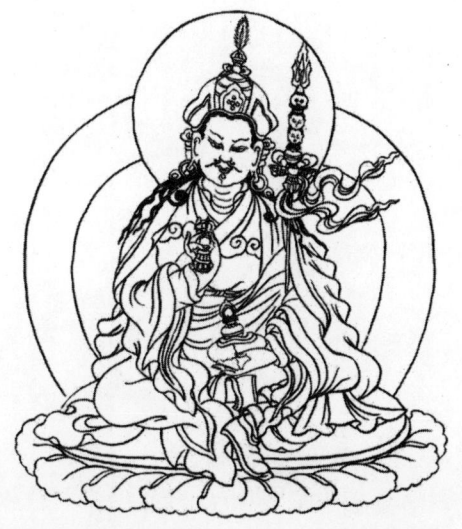

Padmasambhava (Courtesy: www.buddhanet.net)

PART II
ATIYOGA

1. Premise

THIS section contains the commented translation of a Tibetan text that expounds the most essential instructions of the Buddhist Dzogchen (Great Completeness) doctrine, also known in Sanskrit as *Atiyoga* (Extreme Union).[1]

The author is Padmasambhava, the "Lotus-Born," the legendary Buddhist *guru* hailing from an ancient Indian kingdom known as Uḍḍiyāna. Deemed to have been the first to introduce the esoteric teachings of the Tantras into Tibet, he also participated in the foundation of Samye (*bSam yas*) temple, which dates back to 755 CE.

The present text belongs to the same literary cycle that includes the celebrated "Tibetan Book of the Dead." However, instead of prescribing the visualizations, *mantra*s or words of

---

1. *Rig pa ngo sprod gcer mthong rang grol*, in *Zab chos zhi khro dgongs pa rang grol las bar do thos grol gyi skor*, Dharamsala, 1984, vol. tha, pp. 373-402 = A. I have compared the printed edition in my possession with the one belonging to the Tucci Tibetan Fund at IsIAO in Rome (vol. na, ff. 1-25a) = B. Cf. Dieter Michael Back, *Rig pa ṅo sprod gcer mthoṅ raṅ grol. Die Erkenntnislehre des Bar do thosgrol*, Wiesbaden, 1987, pp. 78ff. For other translations cf. W.Y. Evans-Wentz, *The Tibetan Book of the Great Liberation*, London, 1954, pp. 202-39; John Myrdhin Reynolds, *Self-liberation through seeing with naked awareness*, New York, 1989, pp. 71ff; Robert A.F. Thurman, *The Tibetan Book of the Dead*, London, 1994, pp. 227-42.

power, *mudrā*s or symbolic gestures and other characteristic techniques of the Buddhist tāntric methods, it advocates pure awareness (*rig pa*) alone, in which the true natural and original state of the individual and of all of existence reveals itself spontaneously, beyond all mental elaboration and personal striving to attain it.

Padmasambhava's teaching is in the form of a compendium of brief instructions, addressed to Buddhist practitioners to enable them to understand the innermost essence and single goal common to all the innumerable spiritual doctrines and various methods of practice, beyond their apparent or real differences.

The translation of Padmasambhava's text is followed by a commentary by Lama Rangdröl Naljor. I met the Lama in December 1989; at that time he was staying in Delhi, waiting to return to his Himalayan hermitage. I think that it would not have been possible to meet him had Sherab Senge, one of his few Tibetan disciples, not spoken of him to me. The Lama is an elderly Dzogchen master, who, however, dresses as a simple Tibetan layman and spends most of his time in solitary mountain hermitages.

The first time I saw him I brought with me Padmasambhava's text and a revealed scripture (Tantra) known in Tibetan as *Kunje Gyalpo* (*Kun byed rgyal po*), "The Sovereign Creator of All."[2] As soon as he saw me, the Lama asked what I

---

2. *Chos thams cad rdzogs pa chen po byang chub kyi sems kun byed rgyal po*, in *rNying ma'i rgyud 'bum — A Collection of Treasured Tantras Translated During the Period of First Propagation of Buddhism in Tibet*, ed. by Dingo Khyentse Rinpoche, Thimphu, Bhutan, 1973, vol. ka, pp. 1-220 = A; *The mTshams-brag Manuscript of the rNying ma rgyud 'bum*, Thimphu, Bhutan, 1982, vol. ka, pp. 1-261 = B; in *The Tibetan Tripitaka*, Tokyo-Kyoto, 1956, No. 451, vol. dza/9, pp. 93-126 = C. Cf. E. K. Neumaier-Dargay, *The Sovereign All-Creating Mind — The Motherly Buddha*, Albany, 1992; Chögyal Namkhai Norbu, Adriano Clemente, trans. Andrew Lukianowicz, *The Supreme Source*, Ithaca, 1999; Longchenpa, trans. Kennard Lipman and Merrill Peterson, *You Are the Eyes of the World*, Novato, 1987.

Premise

was doing with those Tibetan books. Somewhat embarrassed, I explained that I intended to translate the text by Padmasambhava and to study the Tantra, as I knew it was a fundamental source of the Dzogchen teaching.

The Lama remained still, silently watching me for a few seconds, then stretched out both hands and asked for the texts. He stayed rapt for a while, looking at them without opening them, then he placed the texts on my head one at a time, chanting some verses in Tibetan, and told me that this simple rite was their transmission. He then opened the text by Padmasambhava and started explaining it, quoting by heart several passages from the *Kunje Gyalpo* Tantra.

2. The Introduction to Awareness

Homage to the three-bodied deity,
self-resplendent awareness!

> From "The Profound Teaching
> on Natural Liberation
> through Contemplation
> on the Peaceful and Wrathful Deities:"
>
> The Introduction to Awareness
> Natural Liberation through Seeing Nakedly

CONTEMPLATE well by means of the introduction to self-awareness here expounded. O worthy sons! *Samayā*. Sealed, sealed, sealed.

Oh! The single consciousness that pervades both transmigration and liberation is actually ourselves from the very beginning, yet we do not recognize it; its clear awareness is unceasing, yet we do not encounter it; it appears everywhere without obstacles, yet we do not discern it.

In order to be able to recognize our true nature, there is nothing within the countless teachings of the victorious ones of the three times, such as the 84,000 doors of the *Dharma*, that goes beyond this understanding.

The Introduction to Awareness

Even though the sacred scriptures are infinite as the expanse of the sky, in conclusion their meaning is the introduction to awareness, expressible in three words. Direct introduction to the intention of the victorious ones is precisely this teaching, indicated without secrecy.

O worthy sons, listen to me!

The word "consciousness" is well known, but how many limited assertions have arisen from misconstruing it, from erroneous or partial knowledge of it and from misunderstanding its real meaning.

Common individuals, who do not understand their true nature, wander among the six beings of the three worlds undergoing suffering; this is the defect of misconstruing one's consciousness as it is in itself.

Those who follow extremist doctrines have erroneous understanding because they fall within the limits of permanence and cessation.

The understanding of the hearers and of the spontaneous victors is only partial; they affirm that they understand the absence of ego but their understanding is not perfect. Moreover, they do not contemplate the clear light because they are conditioned by their philosophical positions and by their authoritative texts. In fact, the hearers and the spontaneous victors are hindered by attachment to object and subject.

The followers of the "middle way" are hindered by attachment to their conception of the two truths.

The followers [of the Tantras] of ritual action, [the twofold ones] and [those] of union are hindered by attachment to their conception of the phases of worship.

The followers [of the Tantras] of great union and of subsequent union are hindered by attachment to their conception of the source and of awareness.

They go astray because they divide into two that which is devoid of duality; not attaining the unity in which there is no duality, they do not accomplish enlightenment.

In the consciousness of all [beings] there is no separation between transmigration and liberation, so due to these vehicles that entail rejection and assent, renunciation and acceptance, [beings] continue to wander in transmigration.

The three bodies [of the Buddhas] are naturally present, without any effort, in self-awareness; nevertheless, fools who make calculations about levels and paths through methods for going far, towards something else that is not this [truth], are indolent regarding the [definitive] meaning.

The Buddhas' state of consciousness is beyond the mind, nevertheless, those who meditate on specific images and practise the recitation [of *mantra*s] deceive themselves [regarding this truth].

Thus, you must leave everything, remaining free of any altering action. Then, thanks to this teaching on natural liberation through seeing awareness nakedly you should understand that all reality abides in great natural liberation, so everything is also complete in the state of Great Completeness. *Samayā*. Sealed, sealed, sealed.

Oh! The limpid awareness that we call "consciousness" does not exist as something [concrete, yet] from it all the suffering and happiness of transmigration and liberation arise; conceived according to the beliefs of the eleven vehicles, it has countless different names. Some say it is the true nature of consciousness. Some non-Buddhists call it the "self." The hearers say it is the absence of a personal ego. The idealists call it "consciousness." Some call it the "middle way." Some say it is transcendent knowledge. Some call it the "essence of the realized beings." Some call it "great seal." Some call it the "single point." Some call it the "source of reality." Some call it "universal base." Some call it "ordinary feeling."

The Introduction to Awareness

Should [the master] introduce [awareness] pointing directly just to it [the instruction is as follows].

After the past thought has faded without leaving a trace and the future thought has not yet arisen, [the mind] is fresh and as new. In this moment, while observing yourself nakedly, remaining natural in the present without creating anything, the ordinary, common, everyday feeling is clarity in which there is nothing to see; it is limpidity in which awareness is evident and naked; it is a pure and empty state in which there is nothing that can be determined; it is lucidity in which clarity and emptiness are not two.

It is not something permanent, in fact in no way can it be determined; nor is it nothing, because it is a state of limpid clarity. It is not single inasmuch as it is clear awareness in multiplicity; nor can it be determined as multiple, because it is the one taste of inseparability. It is not extrinsic, it is just self-awareness.

This being the actual introduction to the true nature of reality, here the three bodies [of the Buddhas] are inseparably complete in unity. Emptiness, nothing determinable, is the reality body; clarity, the natural splendour of emptiness, is the fruition body; the manifestation appearing everywhere without obstacles is the emanation body. The completeness of the three bodies in unity is the essential state.

Should [the master] introduce [awareness] instantaneously pointing just to it [the instruction is as follows].

It is just feeling yourself in the present moment; it is just this unaltered and self-resplendent state. Why, then, do you say you don't understand the true nature of consciousness? Here there is nothing on which to meditate. Why, then, do you say that, even meditating, it does not appear?

It is just this immediate awareness. Why, then, do you say you do not find your own consciousness? It is just this unceasing clear awareness. Why, then, do you say you do not see the face of consciousness? It is just the thinker. Why, then, do you say that, even seeking it, you do not find it?

Here there is nothing to do. Why, then, do you say that, even though you do [the practice], it does not appear? Remaining in your state, without modifying it, is enough. Why, then, do you say you cannot stay in it? Remaining as you are, without doing anything, is enough. Why, then, do you say you have not the strength to do it?

Emptiness, clarity and awareness are inseparable and spontaneously present. Why, then, do you say that, even engaging in it, you do not realize yourself? Spontaneously arising, without causes or conditions, it exists spontaneously. Why, then, do you say that, even striving, you are not able [to realize it]?

Thoughts arise and dissolve at the same time. Why, then, do you say you cannot free yourself [of them] by applying an antidote? It is just this feeling of the present moment. Why, then, do you say you do not know it?

The true nature of consciousness is certainly empty and without a base; it is not concrete, like empty space. Contemplate your own consciousness to understand if this is really so.

This is not the emptiness of the nihilist view, in fact spontaneous knowledge is certainly radiant from the very beginning; it is self-arising and self-resplendent like the heart of the sun. Contemplate your own consciousness to understand if this is really so.

Awareness is certainly unceasing from the very beginning; it is like the main current of a river that flows continuously. Contemplate your own consciousness to understand if this is really so.

Mental fluctuations certainly cannot be grasped; they are movements without solidity like a breeze in the sky. Contemplate your own consciousness to understand if this is really so.

All phenomena, whatever they are, are certainly our own manifestation; whatever appears is like our reflection in a mirror. Contemplate your own consciousness to understand if this is really so.

All [mental] images certainly dissolve spontaneously; they arise by themselves and dissolve by themselves like clouds in the sky. Contemplate your own consciousness to understand if this is really so.

There is nothing but consciousness; apart from this there is no view from which to observe. There is nothing but consciousness; apart from this there is no meditation to practise. There is nothing but consciousness; apart from this there is no conduct to apply. There is nothing but consciousness; apart from this there is no commitment to keep. There is nothing but consciousness; apart from this there is no goal to realize.

Contemplate often, contemplate your own consciousness. Observing outwards, out in celestial space, there is no place towards which consciousness moves. Observing inwards, here inside your own consciousness, there is no one who moves with thought. Hence, your own consciousness is luminously resplendent without sparkling.

The clear light of self-awareness is empty, [so] it is the reality body; like the sun arising in a bright cloudless sky, it knows every thing clearly but without any concepts. There is a great difference between understanding it and not understanding it.

Incredible! This clear light, unborn from the very beginning and natural, is awareness, the young child without father or mother. Not produced by anybody, it is spontaneous knowledge. Not having experienced birth, it does not die.

Incredible! Although it shines directly, there is no observer. Even though one wanders in transmigration, it does not become something bad. Even though one attains liberation, it does not become something good.

Incredible! Although it exists everywhere, it is not understood. [Even though it is] the goal, people neglect it, wishing for another goal. Even though it is oneself, people seek it elsewhere.

Marvellous!

This awareness of the present moment, indeterminable and clear, is indeed the utmost peak of all views.

Without an image as support, omnipresent, not bound by the mind, it is indeed the utmost peak of all meditations.

This unaltered state of relaxation without any attachment is indeed the utmost peak of all conducts.

This realization, innate from the very beginning and not sought at all, is indeed the utmost peak of all goals.

I will explain the four great straight threads.

The great thread of right view is this limpid feeling of the present moment; it is called "thread" because it is clear and does not allow errors.

The great thread of right meditation is this limpid feeling of the present moment; it is called "thread" because it is clear and does not allow errors.

The great thread of right conduct is this limpid feeling of the present moment; it is called "thread" because it is clear and does not allow errors.

The great thread of the right goal is this limpid feeling of the present moment; it is called "thread" because it is clear and does not allow errors.

I will explain the four great firm nails.

The great nail of the unchanging view is just this limpid feeling of the present moment; it is called "nail" because it is stable in the three times.

The Introduction to Awareness

The great nail of unchanging meditation is just this limpid feeling of the present moment; it is called "nail" because it is stable in the three times.

The great nail of unchanging conduct is just this limpid feeling of the present moment; it is called "nail" because it is stable in the three times.

The great nail of the unchanging goal is just this limpid feeling of the present moment; it is called "nail" because it is stable in the three times.

Here is the instruction that enables you to abide in the unity of the three times.

Not attending to the past, leave any considerations about what has passed; not anticipating the future, cut the bonds of mental associations; not grasping the present, remain in the condition of space.

As there is nothing on which to meditate, do not meditate on anything, and as there is no reason to get distracted, rely on undistracted presence. Without meditating, without getting distracted, simply observe.

Self-awareness, feeling oneself that arises limpidly and shines by its own light, is enlightened consciousness. There is nothing on which to meditate, in fact it is beyond the knowable; there is no distraction, in fact it is clear by nature. Empty phenomena resolve themselves spontaneously, and empty clarity is the reality body.

As it is the manifestation of enlightenment not realized by means of a path it is the vision of Diamond Being in this very moment.

Here is the teaching on the definitive consumption.

Although there are countless conflicting views, in spontaneous knowledge, in the true nature of self-aware consciousness, there is no duality of observer and observed.

Do not have a point of view, [rather] seek the observer. When, seeking the observer, you do not find the observer, then the view has been consumed; right here you also achieve the final view.

There is no point of view from which to observe; however, without falling into nihilist indifference, limpid feeling oneself in the present moment is the view of the great understanding. Here there is no duality of understanding and not understanding.

Although there are countless conflicting meditations, in the omnipresent ordinary feeling of self-awareness there is no duality of meditation and meditator.

Do not meditate, [rather] seek the meditator. When, seeking the meditator, you do not find the meditator, then meditation has been consumed; right here you also achieve the final meditation.

There is no meditation to engage; however, without letting yourself be overcome by the various forms of torpor and agitation, clear unaltered feeling of the present moment is contemplation of the even and uncontrived state. Here there is no dualism of calm and agitation.

Although there are countless conflicting conducts, in the single point of self-aware knowledge there is no duality of conduct and one who applies it.

Do not practise a conduct, [rather] seek the one who is practising it. When, seeking the one who is practising it, you do not find its practitioner, then the conduct has been consumed; right here you also achieve the final conduct.

There is no conduct to apply; however, without letting yourself be conditioned by the illusion of latent tendencies, the feeling of the present moment, unaltered and self-resplendent, in which there is nothing to correct, modify, obtain or give up, is itself absolutely pure conduct. Here there is no duality of pure and impure.

The Introduction to Awareness

Although there are countless conflicting goals, in the true nature of self-aware consciousness the three bodies [of the Buddhas] are an innate realization. Here there is no duality of realization and the one who realizes.

Do not seek to realize the goal, [rather] seek just the one who realizes it. When, seeking the one who realizes it, you do not find him or her, then the goal has been consumed; right here you also achieve the final goal.

There is no goal to realize; however, without letting yourself be conditioned by rejection and obtainment, by hope and fear, understand that the self-replendent feeling of the present moment is innate realization, because here, within oneself, the three bodies are fully manifest; precisely this is the goal of original enlightenment.

This awareness, unbound by the eight limits of permanence and cessation [etc.], is called the "middle way" inasmuch as it does not fall into those extremes. It is called "awareness" because presence is unceasing. It is given the name "essence of the realized beings" because it is emptiness that has the nature of awareness.

When there is this understanding one transcends all the knowable, thus it is also called "transcendent knowledge." Beyond the mind, from the very beginning it is not bound by the extremes of conclusions, so it is given the name "great seal."

Due to the difference between understanding it and not understanding it, it becomes the basis of all the happiness and suffering of liberation and transmigration so that it is called "universal base." Just this ordinary, common, everyday feeling, clear and limpid, is given the name "ordinary feeling."

However many pleasant names and beautiful definitions there may be, really whoever aspires to something more, to something different from this feeling of the present moment, is like someone who follows the footsteps of an elephant in spite of having already found it. Even if he follows [its footsteps] in the numerous worlds, he will never find [the elephant]; in the same way, aside from consciousness enlightenment can never be found.

Not having understood it, one seeks consciousness outside; however, how can one find oneself by seeking oneself in what is other than oneself? It is like an idiot giving up his own identity in order to mimic many people and, subsequently, no longer recognizing himself, looking for himself elsewhere and confusing himself with someone else.

Not seeing the real condition of things, we do not understand that phenomena are consciousness, so we deviate into transmigration. Not understanding that enlightenment is our own consciousness, liberation is obscured.

Transmigration and liberation are no more different from each other than understanding and not understanding are in their single instant; we are deluded when we see them as other than our own consciousness.

Illusion and disillusion are of one essence; in a being there are not two threads of consciousness, so illusion dissolves when we leave consciousness itself in its own unaltered natural state.

When not aware of the fact that illusion itself is consciousness, not understanding at all the true nature of reality, you should observe by yourself and within yourself that which arises spontaneously.

At the beginning, whence do these phenomena arise? Then, where do they abide? Finally, where do they vanish? Observe them as if they were crows on a boat [in the middle of the sea]; they fly off from the boat but they have no other place to alight. In the same way, phenomena arise from consciousness and dissolve in it.

The true nature of consciousness, empty clarity that feels everything and is aware of everything, is like space in which clarity and emptiness are inseparable from the beginning.

The Introduction to Awareness

Ascertaining clearly and directly that it is spontaneous knowledge, this itself is the real condition. Here is the proof: you understand that all phenomena are consciousness and that the nature of consciousness, being clear awareness, is like space.

Although the example of space is used to point out the real condition, it is only a symbol that indicates it partially. The nature of consciousness is endowed with awareness, an emptiness that is utterly clear; space is unaware, an emptiness devoid of matter. This is the reason why the nature of consciousness cannot really be indicated by [the example of] space. Remain in the condition [of space] without getting distracted.

One cannot demonstrate the real existence of any of the diverse phenomena as they appear conventionally; in fact they disappear.

To exemplify that, [consider] all reality, transmigration and liberation, to be only the manifestation of your own consciousness. When [your] state of consciousness changes the corresponding manifestation appears externally.

Thus, everything is a manifestation of consciousness. The six kinds of common beings hold distinct views of phenomena; outside [Buddhism], the extremists hold the dualistic view of permanence and cessation; and the nine levels of vehicles hold distinct views.

You see various things and various things are not the same; so, as you grasp the differences, you are beguiled by personal attachment. When you are aware that all phenomena are consciousness, even though the perception of phenomena arises, by not grasping [it] you are Buddha.

It is not phenomena that beguile, it is grasping them that beguiles. Grasping dissolves by itself when you are aware that it is consciousness.

Whatever appears is a manifestation of consciousness. The material vision of the external world, too, is consciousness.

What appears as the six kinds of common beings, too, is consciousness; the beatific vision of the deities in their worlds and of humans is consciousness, and the painful vision of the three lower worlds is consciousness.

What appears as the five emotional poisons, that is misunderstanding [and the other poisons], is consciousness and what appears as the awareness of spontaneous knowledge, too, is consciousness.

What appears as the latent traces of transmigration [determined by] negative thoughts is consciousness and what appears as the heavens of liberation [determined by] positive thoughts is consciousness.

What appears as the obstacles of demons and evil forces is consciousness and what appears benign, such as deities and realizations, is consciousness.

What appears as various concepts is consciousness and what appears as the non-conceptual state of concentration, too, is consciousness.

What appears as the colour that characterizes things is consciousness and what appears as simple and devoid of characteristics, too, is consciousness.

What appears as free of the dichotomy of unity and multiplicity is consciousness and what appears as utterly indeterminable as regards existence and non-existence, too, is consciousness.

There is no phenomenon that is not consciousness. Whatever phenomenon appears [by virtue of] the unhindered nature of consciousness, although it arises, is like a wave in relation to the ocean; as there is no duality it resolves itself in consciousness itself.

Even though names are given due to the free presence of what is to be named, whatever the name is [that indicates authentic reality], in truth there is nothing but single consciousness; moreover, it is without a base, without a root.

There is no unilateral point of view. Do not hold a concrete view because [consciousness] cannot be determined at all; do not hold the view of emptiness because there is the splendour of clear awareness; do not hold a fragmentary view because clarity and emptiness are inseparable.

Although feeling oneself in the present moment is clear and limpid, you do not know who it is that makes it so. It is impersonal, yet it can be experienced directly.

All [beings] can liberate themselves by experiencing this state [of pure awareness]. In fact, its recognition happens without any difference regarding the capacity [of understanding], whether it is sharp or dull.

Even though sesame and milk are the causes of oil and butter, if sesame is not ground and milk not churned there will be neither oil nor butter. Actually, all beings are potential Buddhas, but if they do not experience [awareness of their own true nature] they do not get enlightened, whereas even a herdsman gets liberated by experiencing it.

Although one does not know how to explain it, it can be ascertained directly; it is like tasting sugar so that you no longer need someone else to explain its flavour.

Even great scholars are subject to delusion if they do not have this understanding. You can become expert in the field of the nine vehicles but it is like recounting a tale about something far away that you have never seen; in this way you do not approach enlightenment at all.

If you have this understanding, virtue and vice dissolve spontaneously; if it is lacking, then whatever action you perform, whether it is virtuous or not, you will not transcend transmigration in the upper or lower worlds.

As soon as you understand the knowledge of your empty and clear consciousness there is no longer any real positive or negative consequence of virtuous or vicious actions. Just as a river does not gush out of empty space, so virtue and vice do not objectively exist in emptiness.

Thus, to see directly self-awareness in its nakedness, this teaching on natural liberation through seeing nakedly is really profound, so right here is where you must examine what self-awareness is. Deeply sealed.

Marvellous! This introduction to awareness, natural liberation through seeing nakedly, is a brief and clear synthesis composed taking into account the sacred scriptures, the revealed messages, the teachings of the masters and personal experience, with the aspiration to benefit the worthy ones of the dark age, those of future generations. At this time [the text] cannot be propagated; let it be concealed as a precious treasure. In future let it be discovered by the person destined to do so. *Samayā*. Sealed, sealed, sealed.

This text on direct introduction to awareness, called "Natural Liberation through Seeing Nakedly," was composed by Padmasambhava, Abbot of Uḍḍiyāna. May [this teaching] not end until transmigration has been emptied.

3. Commentary

Homage to the three-bodied deity,
self-resplendent awareness!

WHY do you ask me for what is already in you from the very beginning? Let go of your search for erudition. Stop investigating with your mind. The only thing necessary is to let our true nature disclose itself and show us what we have always been.

Which is your deity? Who or what is your refuge? This teaching says that the supreme deity, the true refuge, is awareness, full consciousness of what we really are, beyond all mental convictions. Such awareness does not come from outside but from within us. Outer reality is only a mirror in which we can see our own face. As long as we seek outside ourselves we will never find the true meaning of our existence. The source of the light that makes appear and illuminates the outside as well as the inside has always been within us; that is where we should seek the supreme deity.

So, the authentic spiritual tradition cannot be received from outside because it originates only from the enlightened consciousness that we have within us; even the book that contains this tradition is solely a mirror, reflecting what is already present within us. In fact, the words of the deity, revealed in the *Kunje Gyalpo* Tantra, symbolize the way in which enlightened consciousness reveals itself to itself in the limpid emptiness of our being:

1. O Great Diamond Being, listen! From the very beginning, I am spontaneous knowledge. From the very beginning, I am the matrix of all reality. I am enlightened consciousness, the sovereign creator of all. [You Great] Being, understand my name; if [you Great] Being understand it, then [you] will also understand all of reality.

What do these mysterious expressions of the Tantra mean? Enlightened consciousness itself makes their meaning clear within us:

2. The term "I" means the matrix, because I am the matrix of all reality. "Spontaneous" refers to the matrix inasmuch as it is without cause or conditions and, thus, it is beyond all effort. "Knowledge" signifies what reveals every thing because it is without obstacles or obscuration. I am called enlightened consciousness. "From the very beginning" means that I have been present from the very origin.

The expression "all reality" stands for all the masters, their teachings and also those who receive them, the places where they are transmitted and the times of the transmission; reality embraces everything. The "matrix" is the source whence everything issues; in fact, it is from the natural state of enlightened consciousness that there appear the three masters, their teachings and also those who receive them, the places and the times of the transmission.

I, the matrix, the true nature of consciousness, am the creator of all. [. . .] The creator is the maker; having created all, that is the masters, the teachings, those who receive them, the places and times, spontaneous knowledge is the creator. The matrix, spontaneous knowledge, is said to be "sovereign" because the creator is above all: the maker of reality is the universal monarch.

["Enlightened" means pure and total.] "Pure" refers to the fact that being spontaneous, enlightened consciousness, the matrix is pure from the very beginning, so everything created by the sovereign creator of all is utterly pure like [the Primordial Buddha] Universal Goodness himself. It is said to be "total" because spontaneous knowledge, the matrix, including all reality (animate and inanimate, the environment and those who live in it, the Buddhas of the three times, the beings of the six families in the three worlds and every thing) is omnipresent. "Consciousness" stands for spontaneous knowledge, the matrix that is present in all reality governing and establishing every thing clearly. This matrix which is without cause and conditions, and governs every thing, is the creator of all.

Great Being, if you understand my natural state you will also understand all the masters, their teachings, the thoughts of their disciples and also the places and times of the transmissions, because all is one. All that exists is me, so, if you understand my natural state you will understand all that is and, without effort, you will spontaneously realize that which is beyond doer, deed and all striving.

All these words only serve to indicate the Buddhas' three bodies, that correspond to essence, existence and grace, the three aspects of enlightened consciousness:

3. My unaltered essence is realized as the reality body; my unaltered existence is the complete fruition body; my manifest grace is the emanation body.

In what do the three bodies of the Primordial Buddha, here called "Universal Goodness," consist? In emptiness or the absence of dualistic concepts, clarity or the presence of phenomena, and the free expression of natural wisdom:[1]

4. I am enlightened consciousness, the lamp of the masters; I am the matrix of the Buddhas of the three times; I am the father and mother of the beings of the three worlds; I am also

---

1. Natural wisdom (*rang 'byung ye shes*) is the manifestation of the single spontaneous knowledge through the manifold experiences of the various emotions. See note 14.

the cause of all reality, the environment and those who live in it. There is nothing that does not come forth from me.

I have no abode, I am immanent in everything, so, from the very beginning I am the Buddhas of the three times. Since I remain in equanimity without creating dualistic concepts I am the Primordial Buddha in the reality body, even and free of images. Since my existence is enjoyed everywhere, I am the Primordial Buddha in the complete fruition body. Since I appear as natural wisdom, I am the Buddha manifest in the emanation body [that constitutes my] grace.

Thus, the physical body, voice and spirit of the supreme deity are none other than the forms, sounds and indeterminable state of being of all that is:

5. I have no existence constituting my physical body other than what appears as the outer environment and the beings living within it; thus, the master that teaches is the very existence [of things].

[. . .] I have no voice other than the sounds of all beings and those of earth, water, fire, air and ether; thus, the teaching is given by ascribing meaning to sounds.

[. . .] I have no spirit other than the even and non-conceptual state [of the essence], the true nature of reality, unborn, devoid of images and without obstacles, proper to all beings and to the five elements.

Even the words designating the three fundamental aspects or seals of enlightened consciousness merely indicate the single word that points straight to our own heart, to the unaltered and indeterminable matrix, to the spontaneous knowledge of awareness:

6. In the sovereign master that is the creator of all, I who am the spontaneous knowledge of awareness, the three masters too converge. [. . .] The three teachings too converge and remain in the teaching of awareness beyond words and symbols. The three abodes too converge in the supreme abode of unaltered awareness. All phenomena converge in the matrix,

enlightened consciousness, thus the three kinds of disciples and the three times too converge in it. There is nothing beyond the knowledge in which all converge.

Therefore, true homage, supreme worship, is beyond words and concepts, in the same way that naked awareness is. If you have understood this, no other words are necessary.

RANGDRÖL NALJOR (RN): Do you want to ask me any questions?

GIUSEPPE BAROETTO (GB): Yes. It seems to me that the concept of "enlightened consciousness" revealed in the Tantras is not the same as that found in the Sūtras. Is that the case?

RN: The esoteric concept found in the Tantras includes and transcends the common one of the Sūtras. The Sūtras teach that, on the relative plane, enlightened consciousness is one's aspiration and the consequent actual commitment that all beings realize the state of Buddha. In the absolute sense, enlightened consciousness is both the awareness realized by Buddha and the pure essence that constitutes the seed of awakening, innate through all time in all beings.

The Tantras also teach that, on the relative plane, the enlightened consciousness is the creative principle present in the sperm and ovum while, on the absolute plane, it is the supreme deity and the true nature of all reality.

GB: According to you, is the concept of deity revealed in the *Kunje Gyalpo* Tantra in some ways compatible with the theologies of other religions?

RN: It is not up to me to say what correspondences there might be between one religious tradition and another. Find that out for yourself. For me, the supreme deity is the unborn, the unconditioned, freedom from illusion, from egoism and from suffering, and also the ineffable absolute source of all reality, the intelligence that rules over the manifestations of existence and life itself in all its forms.

GB: Why is the emanation body, the grace of the deity, defined as the unhindered expression of natural wisdom?

RN: Grace is the love that connects essence and existence, emptiness and clarity, subject and object; without it life could not express itself. You have manifested in this world and continue to express yourself unhindered, freely, thanks to the grace of love. Wouldn't you agree?

* * *

*From "The Profound Teaching
on Natural Liberation
through Contemplation
on the Peaceful and Wrathful Deities:"*

*The Introduction to Awareness
Natural Liberation through Seeing Nakedly*

Contemplate well by means of the introduction to self-awareness here expounded. O worthy sons! Samayā. *Sealed, sealed, sealed.*

This teaching forms part of a cycle of instructions imparted in Tibet by Padmasambhava, the master from Uḍḍiyāna. Yet, the true "Precious Teacher" (Guru Rinpoche) is not a person who lived over one thousand years ago. Rather he is our true original nature which is identical to that of all other beings, the Great Self (*bdag nyid chen po*), that is free of the images with which individuals identify themselves.

The true peaceful and wrathful deities, too, are not individuals existing separately from ourselves, rather they are manifestations of our own consciousness. We should neither hope for nor fear visions of them; when they appear it is enough to recognise them as symbolic forms taken on by the Self and to maintain our awareness limpid and empty.

During our life, the triple seal of enlightened consciousness should be recognized in every experience. All the beings around us are sacred peaceful or wrathful forms, reflecting

Commentary

our own qualities or defects. Every phenomenon is a signal, a pointer along the path, a message and help from our Self. So, it is important, starting right now, to be able to go beyond hope and fear, attachment and aversion, keeping awareness unperturbed, limpid yet devoid of dualistic concepts.

If you enact the precious advice found in this book, you will be able to understand what naked awareness consists in. When that happens you liberate yourself spontaneously, without alteration or effort, from the chains of conditioning that bind us to the world.

The *samaya*, the commitment undertaken by those who want to put into practice this teaching, is solely to remain aware in our natural state:

7. Self-awareness is the means of knowledge free of errors by which we understand the unaltered matrix [of reality].

This is what the Tantra says. In fact, being present in the present, without altering anything, is precisely the essential method that human beings can apply naturally. All the other methods can be useful, in certain cases, but they are secondary, like branches in relation to the trunk.

RN: Do you have any questions?

GB: I would like to ask you why this teaching does not mention the preliminary practices.

RN: The way taught by Padmasambhava is that of natural liberation, and even if there were only one person in the world able to follow it, then it is well that it be taught correctly, without imposing artificial, corrective methods that would change it into a different path. It is an opportunity offered to those who need it.

GB: Don't you think that the expression "Great Self" matches Buddhism with Hinduism?

RN: Maybe, however it is only a term, its real meaning is our true nature that is unborn and unceasing.

GB: You said that we should deem all beings to be deities. That is not at all easy. Do you consider the Chinese, who have conquered your country, ruthlessly torturing and killing many people, to be wrathful deities?

RN: There was a time when, in my meditation, I recognized the various tyrants in my life as so many wrathful deities. You know, it is thanks to my oppressors that I learned to be completely free and to truly love. If this had not happened you could not have met me. Do you think I would have had the courage to descend from my paradise on the mountain to come into this tumultuous city?

Now I see that all is Kunje Gyalpo, even those that could be considered our worst enemies. We Tibetans are the expression of the divine life just as the Chinese are, so we are mirrors for each other because each can learn from the other. We could all awaken to awareness of the Great Self present in every being. This would be true liberation.

* * *

Oh! The single consciousness that pervades both transmigration and liberation is actually ourselves from the very beginning, yet we do not recognize it; its clear awareness is unceasing, yet we do not encounter it; it appears everywhere without obstacles, yet we do not discern it.

In order to be able to recognize our true nature, there is nothing within the countless teachings of the victorious ones of the three times, such as the 84,000 doors of the Dharma,[2] *that go beyond this understanding.*

---

2. According to the Buddhist scriptures, there are 84,000 misleading thoughts or emotions that veil vision of the ultimate nature, whence there are as many teachings (*Dharma*) for the realization of the full awakening of awareness. The "victorious ones of the three times" are the enlightened beings of the past, present and future.

Commentary

> *Even though the sacred scriptures are infinite as the expanse of the sky, in conclusion their meaning is the introduction to awareness, expressible in three words. Direct introduction to the intention of the victorious ones is precisely this teaching, indicated without secrecy.*

If you believe that your consciousness is really separate and different from that of other beings, then you are deceiving yourself because, really, nothing exists apart from one single impersonal consciousness. Both transmigration, passing from one experience to another, now and after death, life after life, and release from this process of becoming conditioned by illusion are the eternal expression of the selfsame enlightened consciousness.

> 8. From the very beginning, all reality, the Buddhas with their qualities, bodies and wisdom, common beings with their bodies and unconscious inclinations, etc., has the nature of enlightened consciousness. I have not taught the Buddhas of the past, who have come forth from me, that anything exists apart from consciousness; the same applies to the Buddhas of the present and will apply to the Buddhas to come.

Throughout all time enlightened consciousness manifests freely, everywhere and in every way, but who recognises it just as it is?

> 9. Even though I appear in front of everybody, those who gather round the [Buddhas'] three bodies conceive me according to their countless concepts.

Those who let themselves get bewildered by the multiplicity and diversity of religions, or stubbornly grasp one specific tradition and reject the others, have not yet understood that all the spiritual teachings have just one heart, that is the awareness whereby we understand our true nature.

> *O worthy sons, listen to me!*
>
> *The word "consciousness" is well known, but how many limited assertions have arisen from misconstruing it, from erroneous or*

partial knowledge of it and from misunderstanding its real meaning.

Common individuals, who do not understand their true nature, wander among the six beings of the three worlds³ undergoing suffering; this is the defect of misconstruing one's consciousness as it is in itself.

Those who follow extremist doctrines have erroneous understanding because they fall within the limits of permanence and cessation.⁴

The understanding of the hearers and of the spontaneous victors is only partial; they affirm that they understand the absence of ego but their understanding is not perfect. Moreover, they do not contemplate the clear light because they are conditioned by their philosophical positions and by their authoritative texts. In fact, the hearers and the spontaneous victors are hindered by attachment to object and subject.⁵

The followers of the "middle way" are hindered by attachment to their conception of the two truths.⁶

---

3. The six beings are the hell-dwellers, hungry ghosts, animals, humans, demigods and gods. They all live in the world of desire, apart from the highest hosts of the gods who live in the world of form or the world without form.
4. Eternalism (permanence) is the belief in the existence of an eternal personal entity, both divine and human; nihilism (cessation) is the belief that there is no cause and effect relation among the present life, the previous one and the one to follow. According to Buddhist scholars, these are the philosophical beliefs held by the non-Buddhists (*tīrthika*).
5. The hearers (*śrāvaka*) uphold the absolute existence of material atoms and instants of consciousness; the spontaneous victors (*pratyekabuddha*) believe that only instants of consciousness really exist.
6. In this context, the "middle way" stands for a Mahāyāna Buddhist school, based on distinction between the conventional truth of relative reality and the ultimate truth of absolute reality.

> *The followers [of the Tantras] of ritual action, [the twofold ones] and [those] of union are hindered by attachment to their conception of the phases of worship.*[7]
>
> *The followers [of the Tantras] of great union and of subsequent union are hindered by attachment to their conception of the source and of awareness.*[8]

Everybody has enlightened consciousness, it being the seed of spiritual awakening, and all experience it as the simple feeling oneself, but how many let this natural knowledge shine just as it is in itself, beyond what they believe they are or try to be?

Common individuals feel themselves be but, erroneously, identify this natural knowledge with the objects they experience: their body, physical sensations, emotions, mental images and ideas.

Those who consider themselves better than common individuals merely because they follow a traditional religion or some spiritual discipline are completely wrong. All concepts, definitions and conceptual determinations are nothing but mental images. All mental images are just fantasies, toys that are useful for those who need them but which are basically delusive.

Religious paths based upon dualistic concepts are like the branches of a tree. Anyone who wants to reach the top of the tree can use the branches to lean on, but it is the trunk you have to climb. If you stop on a branch you will never get to

---

7. According to the esoteric texts belonging to the tāntric systems known as *kriyā* (ritual action), *ubhaya* (twofold) or *caryā* (ceremonial) and *yoga* (union), worship of a personal and outer deity is crucial.

8. The followers of the Tantras classified as *mahāyoga* (great union) and *anuyoga* (subsequent union) meditate on the deity as the expression of the inseparability that characterizes the source of reality and the knowledge of awareness.

the top, and if you go all the way along the length of the branch you run the risk that it will break.

The most profound and essential teaching concerns the trunk, the path of awareness that leads to the understanding of the definitive meaning. Grasping provisional doctrines is like tarrying on the branches or deviating onto other paths that do not lead to full awakening.

They go astray because they divide into two that which is devoid of duality; not attaining the unity in which there is no duality, they do not accomplish enlightenment.

In the consciousness of all [beings] there is no separation between transmigration and liberation, so due to these vehicles that entail rejection and assent, renunciation and acceptance, [beings] continue to wander in transmigration.

Multiplicity and duality are characteristic of the various phenomena, the different experiences of life, yet this is an illusion because, in reality, everything that exists is one, just like the consciousness whence it comes forth:

10. All reality is one in enlightened consciousness, its root. In the enlightened matrix that constitutes the source of everything, if they are counted, various phenomena, Buddhas and common beings, are but one.

Thus, transmigration is not something fundamentally negative to reject in order to become free from suffering, nor is liberation something to expect or to seek as if it were the effect of your effort. Those who continue to live straining towards an achievement might well be great scholars or ascetics, but they have not yet understood the authentic condition of things:

11. The cause is meditation [based on] a view. Whoever claims to obtain the effect by having meditated does not obtain the result through such meditation. In fact, everything is just as it is. Trying to correct reality as it is, is a great error because it is like mistaking the true for the false.

Commentary

Tibetans transmit many deep teachings classified as *Dzogchen* (Great Completeness) but the real meaning of this term is not a book, a doctrine or a meditation technique. Rather it is full awareness of our true nature, the consciousness that does not separate I and others, cause and effect, transmigration and liberation, because it knows every thing as its own natural expression, beyond the illusion of time:

12. Whoever affirms that there are cause and effect does not possess understanding of the Great Completeness. The affirmation that there are two truths, conventional and ultimate, is an assertion that exceeds on the one side and falls short on the other. In this way one does not understand that which is without duality. The understanding of the Buddhas of the three times does not see any dichotomy because they recognize the natural state as oneness.

Buddha Śākyamuni taught the existence of an "unborn," otherwise there would be no way to elude that which is born, however only few understand the true meaning of this expression.[9] Here is what the revelation says:

13. Understand that the sovereign creator of all is unborn. As the root of all reality is myself, the creator of all, if you understand me as the unborn source you will also understand that all is the unborn source.

The "unborn" is enlightened consciousness free of the limits of time and is also the true nature of everything that exists; thus, words like "creator" and "creation" are merely symbols of a deep truth, which, however, transcends the illusion of time:

14. The three times are one, there is no real distinction. Without before, without after, [all] comes forth from the very beginning.

Thus, even that which characterizes the Buddhas (such as their three bodies) is not the consequence of the strenuous quest for spiritual realization:

---

9. The Lama is probably quoting the most ancient sources such as *Udāna* (VIII, 3) and *Itivuttaka* (II, 2, 43).

15. The three bodies, heart of all the victorious ones, [manifest] from my natural state, spontaneously realized without any seeking at all; my unaltered essence is realized as the reality body; my unaltered existence is the complete fruition body; my manifest grace is the emanation body. This is not the result of realization through seeking.

Then, where is the starting point? Where are the levels of the path and the various practices? Where is the goal?

16. All is created by the sovereign creator from the very beginning, thus there is no travelling along paths, there is no training on levels, there is no keeping of commitments, and there is no meditation according to a view.

Since everything appears through the path of great enlightenment, enlightenment does not proceed towards enlightenment. As there is no level beyond enlightenment towards which to proceed, enlightenment does not train on [the level of] enlightenment. As the very nature of commitments is enlightenment itself, enlightenment does not keep commitments about itself. The true nature of meditation is enlightenment itself, thus it does not have to meditate on itself. The object of the view is enlightenment itself, thus enlightenment does not have a point of view regarding itself. So. . . .

So, Padmasambhava teaches thus:

The three bodies [of the Buddhas] are naturally present, without any effort, in self-awareness; nevertheless, fools who make calculations about levels and paths through methods for going far, towards something else that is not this [truth], are indolent regarding the [definitive] meaning.

Those who follow the secondary paths of the branches or who strive to travel the main path along the trunk could abide peacefully in awareness of their natural state, without doing anything to modify what is. In fact:

17. Not understanding that reality, as it appears, is enlightened consciousness, one will not realize enlightened consciousness by pursuing it through modification. [When] this understanding is lacking, one pursues [enlightened consciousness] through modification, however, even if one were to do that over countless eras one would never encounter the bliss of non-effort. [. . .] Masters who get one to modify what is, although they claim to teach the truth, do not teach the definitive doctrine but rather the provisional one.

And Padmasambhava goes on thus:

The Buddhas' state of consciousness is beyond the mind, nevertheless, those who meditate on specific images and practise the recitation [of mantras] deceive themselves [regarding this truth].

Praying or reciting *mantras*, contemplating sacred images or visualizing them, are meditative practices which, at most, can soothe the mind and even produce unusual, gratifying experiences, but the definitive meaning is beyond these mirages and any form of self-affirmation:

18. Oh, masters that have issued from me have taught everyone through the three bodies, saying: "There is a meditative practice." This doctrine has been given to those who like to meditate on images for their personal satisfaction.

Many will find this difficult to accept. On the other hand, the revelation of original purity and spontaneous realization, of non-action and non-effort, is not suitable to everybody:

19. The purpose [of this teaching] is to enable the worthy practitioner of *Atiyoga* with the destiny to have had faith in me, enlightened consciousness creator of all, through numberless eras, to see that there is no view on which to meditate, that there are no commitments to keep, there are no deeds of power to seek, there are no paths to travel, there are no levels on which to train, there are no cause and effect, there are not the two truths, conventional and ultimate, there is nothing on which to meditate nor anything to realize, the

[enlightened] consciousness is not to develop, there is no antidote [to apply against the emotions]. The purpose is to see the natural state of consciousness creator of all.

Some hold that there is a means of realization superior to others, a special teaching, a particular Oriental tradition given high-sounding titles such as *Atiyoga*, "Extreme Union." However, true *Atiyoga* is not that particular Indo-Tibetan tradition, rather it is the universal knowledge innate in the heart of all human beings. It is not the ninth vehicle, it is the only vehicle because it is nothing other than awareness of one's own natural state:

20. I, the creator of all, have taught one single vehicle; I have not taught the doctrine of realization through seeking.

In fact, the definitive meaning is just the true unaltered natural state of all reality:

21. The meaning of non-action is my natural state, the creator of all, because I have no action to accomplish; in me everything is already accomplished from the very beginning, so I am the true nature of reality devoid of action. Besides my natural state, the true nature of reality, there is no "natural state." What is called the "natural state" is the natural state without alteration.

Diamond Being, do not modify unaltered enlightened consciousness. If you modify it, you will have modified me, the creator of all. All phenomena as they appear are my natural state, the creator of all.

O Diamond Being, listen! Meditating on my immutable natural state you alter it, you modify it. If you try to realize me, I who exist spontaneously from the very beginning, you alter me. Travelling a path to reach me, you do not get to me. Seeking me, you do not realize me. Purifying me, you do not purify me. Do not look at me from a point of view, because there is no object [to see]. Do not try to reach me, because there is no path. Do not purify me, because there is no obscuration. [I am] without fixations, free of reference points, simple, beyond concepts.

Many know this teaching but do not put it into practice, so they do not know how to transmit it to others or are afraid to disclose it even to those who are ready. But enlightened consciousness that governs everything evenly is not limited by anything; so, now that the time has come it will knock down temple walls, the frontiers between nations and cultural and linguistic barriers to proclaim anew the ancient and eternal revelation:

> 22. Everything is one, so everything is complete in me. Because all is complete in me, I who am the Great Completeness, effort and striving according to [the principles of] the view, conduct, deeds of power, commitments and levels and paths are unnecessary, as explained above. Those who do not understand this and engage in striving, contradict what is beyond cause and effect, and since they do not experience the bliss of non-action, they will be tainted with the affliction of effort, not knowing [Great Completeness]. Therefore, [the teaching of] Great Completeness beyond cause and effect cannot be applied by those who are not destined to it, who should practise a teaching according to cause and effect.

And Padmasambhava concludes thus:

> *Thus, you must leave everything, remaining free of any altering action. Then, thanks to this teaching on natural liberation through seeing awareness nakedly you should understand that all reality abides in great natural liberation, so everything is also complete in the state of Great Completeness.* Samayā. *Sealed, sealed, sealed.*

Instead of wanting to jump to the top of the tree, those who are not yet ready for this teaching would do better to get a firm grip on the branches nearest to them, but without forgetting that they, too, are part of the tree.

RN: Is it all clear? Have you got any questions?

GB: What is the difference between the full awareness realized by the Buddhas and the simple feeling oneself that all people experience?

RN: There is no real difference because, in essence, they are the same. The seed contains in embryo the whole plant. In the same way, a Buddha's full awareness is present in the feeling oneself common to all human beings.

GB: If that is the case, then there is not only one way to ripen the seed.

RN: Obviously, there are many valid ways but the dualistic ones, those that separate, can be compared to the branches of a tree. Don't get stuck on the branches, because you are the whole tree. Furthermore, bear in mind that there are many trees, some of the same species as yours, others different, but they all join together sky and earth. When you are your tree, without separating anything, then you are in your natural state.

GB: What do you think of the different levels of spiritual realization?

RN: I see that they exist but they are like the branches of a tree; if you get stuck on them, you run the risk of stopping there, but you are already the whole tree! That is why it is said that the supreme way is pathless, every moment is both the base and the goal. And, do you think the tree strives to grow? Its development occurs spontaneously, and the same applies to you if you abide in your natural state, the single level of enlightened consciousness.

GB: So, the way of awareness, that you have compared to the trunk, should not be something to follow to reach the goal, right?

RN: Sure, because if you try to pursue it, then you are not present in the present. Listen! If you are the tree, how can you climb the tree to reach the top?

GB: Why then did you say that to reach the top you need to climb the trunk?

RN: Because there are some people who want to reach the top remaining perched on a branch.

GB: What happens when you reach the top?

RN: Try to stay there as long as you can or come down to climb up again, until you understand that there is no real tree to climb.

GB: At this point I don't understand why you compared the way of awareness to the trunk.

RN: Because just as boughs depend on the trunk whence they branch off, the secondary paths must all issue from the main way of awareness and lead back to it. Most followers of religions do not understand this principle and so they end up stuck on a branch or they fall to the ground. In that case the secondary paths become deviations.

Do not think of the tree with levels and with spiritual paths as something outside you; it is life itself manifesting naturally, starting from a seed present within you from the beginning.

GB: In my meditation I still engage with words and images; should I relinquish them?

RN: There is nothing to relinquish or adopt. If you are in your natural state there is no problem. If you pose yourself the problem that is because you are not true to yourself.

GB: If there is nothing to relinquish, why is there still talk of natural liberation?

RN: This expression is used for the benefit of those who hold on to the idea of having to accomplish spiritual liberation, to enable them to understand that this takes place naturally, when they stop altering what is. In that moment they are free of the idea of liberation itself.

GB: "Non-action" does not mean stopping doing anything at all, does it?

RN: Of course not! It means not altering, being natural, whole, free of conflicts. You are not natural when you judge yourself on the basis of a belief system and a behaviour model, altering what you really are.

GB: Granted the principle of non-action, why, then, does the Tantra state that every thing is created by enlightened consciousness?

RN: Expressly to persuade people not to act altering what is. When you abide in your natural state, of course you act but without the conflicts and contradictions that arise from altering what is. The Primordial Buddha is called Universal Goodness because he knows all is well. Do you understand?

GB: If all is well, then nothing should change, but life is continuous change. I don't understand how to reconcile the change that evidently takes place with the principle of not correcting.

RN: Evidently existence changes, as the manifestation of consciousness is free, however the essence is immutable like celestial space. When we get stuck on a form of change, forgetting the essence, in reality we block change itself in that very form, such that consciousness can no longer express itself freely. This is the cause of suffering, warning us of the stagnation of energy. So, the problem lies in the fact that we identify ourselves to such a degree with what changes that we forget that which does not change, and end up judging every thing as it illusorily appears to us.

Some are convinced that realization is outside them and become so insecure that they feel unworthy of it or feel that they are failures. Conversely, there are also others who create such a superior self-image that they feel entitled to dominate others. All of this means "altering what is." Not altering, not modifying what is, means living in the present moment and really loving, as the Primordial Buddha does, free of guilt feelings, of fear, of doubts and of divisive judgements.

* * *

Commentary

> *Oh! The limpid awareness that we call 'consciousness' does not exist as something [concrete, yet] from it all the suffering and happiness of transmigration and liberation arise; conceived according to the beliefs of the eleven vehicles,[10] it has countless different names. Some say it is the true nature of consciousness. Some non-Buddhists call it the "self." The hearers say it is the absence of a personal ego. The idealists call it "consciousness." Some call it the "middle way." Some say it is transcendent knowledge. Some call it the "essence of the realized beings." Some call it "great seal." Some call it the "single point." Some call it the "source of reality." Some call it "universal base." Some call it "ordinary feeling."*

In sacred texts, various terms recur to indicate a single reality. Many persons have not understood this principle and have thus ended up setting their own tradition against others merely because their labels are different. Truth is not diverse but humans have the defect of differentiating it, getting stuck on the names, definitions, rituals and rules that differ according to cultural conditioning and personal needs:

23. It is on account of different people's beliefs that names are given to my single natural state, creator of all. Some call it enlightened consciousness, or the source of reality, the condition of space, spontaneous knowledge, the reality body, complete fruition body, emanation body, or, also, physical body, voice and spirit [of the Buddhas], omniscience, the All, the five, four or three wisdoms, or, also, source and knowledge. These [names] are given to the single reality, spontaneous enlightened consciousness. They represent the measure of how [people] see me, I who am spontaneous.

Padmasambhava's words are indeed precious because they arise from direct experience, ascertained in the light of sacred texts and of tradition:

---

10. According to an ancient tradition, the ninth vehicle or means (*yāna*) of spiritual realization subsumes three vehicles called *ati*, *spyi ti* and *yang ti*.

Should [the master] introduce [awareness] pointing directly just to it [the instruction is as follows].

After the past thought has faded without leaving a trace and the future thought has not yet arisen, [the mind] is fresh and as new. In this moment, while observing yourself nakedly, remaining natural in the present without creating anything, the ordinary, common, everyday feeling is clarity in which there is nothing to see; it is limpidity in which awareness is evident and naked; it is a pure and empty state in which there is nothing that can be determined; it is lucidity in which clarity and emptiness are not two.

It is not something permanent, in fact in no way can it be determined; nor is it nothing, because it is a state of limpid clarity. It is not single inasmuch as it is clear awareness in multiplicity; nor can it be determined as multiple, because it is the one state of inseparability. It is not extrinsic, it is just self-awareness.

This being the actual introduction to the true nature of reality, here the three bodies [of the Buddhas] are inseparably complete in unity. Emptiness, nothing determinable, is the reality body; clarity, the natural splendour of emptiness, is the fruition body; the manifestation appearing everywhere without obstacles is the emanation body. The completeness of the three bodies in unity is the essential state.

According to the first introduction, the true nature of consciousness reveals itself by itself to itself in the gap between one thought and the next. Naked awareness shines in that mysterious empty space. It precedes concepts, mental images, emotions, words and identification with forms and action, yet it exists also when all these psychophysical functions manifest.

Other teachings ascribe great importance to the sitting posture to assume and hold during meditation (legs crossed, torso perfectly erect, hands one on top of the other in the lap, tongue set against the palate, gaze still, etc.). All this can prove

Commentary

useful, above all to beginners, but it can also become an obstacle if it produces tension, rigidity and dependence. That is why the Tantra often bids us not to correct anything.

There is no rule to observe concerning the posture, nor need you seek deliberately to empty the mind. Remaining where you are, as you are, is enough. The important thing is to relax deeply, letting thoughts arise and disappear naturally, yet without losing awareness:

24. O Diamond Being, contemplate reality as it is!

> While observing thought spontaneously resolving itself, resting in the natural state without distraction there is no forced action; in this way everything appears and resolves itself spontaneously.
>
> O Diamond Being, contemplate reality as it is!
>
> Do not correct your body, do not control the senses and do not remain dumb; there is nothing to do by means of effort. Wherever you let the mind go, rest in the state in which you are not disturbed [by anything].

Here is the fundamental principle that should never be forgotten. Once you have understood it, there is no need for anything else. In fact, all the qualities of the enlightened ones come forth from naked awareness and are comprised within it from the very beginning. Thus, even the three bodies of the Buddhas should not be sought by striving, in the hope of realizing them sooner or later. They are naturally present right here and now. If you remain in silence some time you will be able to confirm the teaching for yourself. . . .

RN: Now ask any questions you may have.

GB: It seems to me that experiencing awareness between two thoughts can vary according to the depth of one's concentration. Is that so?

RN: Naked awareness is like the thread of a pearl necklace. The many thoughts, emotions, sensations and experiences are like the pearls. Without the thread there would be no necklace, and likewise without awareness there could be neither transmigration nor liberation, because life would not manifest but would remain present in potentiality in the treasury of the universal base like a seed in the sky. So, do not discriminate between one state of consciousness and another, as the whole necklace is the precious ornament of your life.

GB: Then, what is the point of considering the space between two thoughts?

RN: It serves to understand that our true nature is continuous awareness that sustains every experience without being conditioned by it. Listen! The necklace is made up of the thread as well as the pearls, so it makes no sense to take one and leave the others. Yet, most people only want the pearls while others seek the thread, putting aside the pearls, and yet others who think they have discovered the thread get stuck there so that they are no longer able to understand the value of every experience.

Why is it taught that consciousness is like the sea, and the water of its calm depths is the same as the turbulent waves? Because, in reality, the substance of spontaneous knowledge is the same as that of the various thoughts. In fact, the awareness between two thoughts is still a thought, the thought of the I (*ngar 'dzin rnam rtog*) in its natural state, unaltered and unlimited.

* * *

Should [the master] introduce [awareness] instantaneously pointing just to it [the instruction is as follows].

It is just feeling yourself in the present moment; it is just this unaltered and self-resplendent state. Why, then, do you say you don't understand the true nature of consciousness? Here there is nothing on which to meditate. Why, then, do you say that, even meditating, it does not appear?

It is just this immediate awareness. Why, then, do you say you do not find your own consciousness? It is just this unceasing clear awareness. Why, then, do you say you do not see the face of consciousness? It is just the thinker. Why, then, do you say that, even seeking it, you do not find it?

Here there is nothing to do. Why, then, do you say that, even though you do [the practice], it does not appear? Remaining in your state, without modifying it, is enough. Why, then, do you say you cannot stay in it? Remaining as you are, without doing anything, is enough. Why, then, do you say you have not the strength to do it?

Emptiness, clarity and awareness are inseparable and spontaneously present. Why, then, do you say that, even engaging in it, you do not realize yourself? Spontaneously arising, without causes or conditions, it exists spontaneously. Why, then, do you say that, even striving, you are not able [to realize it]?

Thoughts arise and dissolve at the same time. Why, then, do you say you cannot free yourself [of them] by applying an antidote? It is just this feeling of the present moment. Why, then, do you say you do not know it?

The second introduction to awareness consists in pointing out the true nature of consciousness directly in the feeling oneself that all humans can experience naturally, in any moment and situation of everyday life.

The human mind is so conditioned to operating by striving, projecting itself outside itself, that, paradoxically, the easiest thing appears the most difficult. Our true nature is utter simplicity, our original state; yet, continuous distraction, disordered habits, accumulated notions, fears and hopes make it appear something complicated, far away in time or even outside ourselves:

25. The view of the Great Completeness, on which you need not meditate, is the quality of my consciousness, creator of all. Due to this great quality of enlightened consciousness the asceticism of effort and engagement is not necessary at all. Being without cause and conditions, it need not be sought.

The state of the goal need not be obtained from someone else. The true nature of reality is yourself, so practising meditation is unnecessary. As [phenomena are] unborn, there is no antidote to make them stop. Do not pay attention to anything else. Do not seek the place of meditation. Whoever meditates on me will not meet me, precisely because of the meditation.

As the reality that manifests is me, pain does not arise and it is not necessary to reject anything. Being spontaneous, I am neither born nor do I die, so it is not necessary to suspend sensory [and mental] functions [in order to interrupt] the chain of causation [that starts with] ignorance.

In order not to have any doubt regarding the real meaning of the instruction, there are some explanations using symbols. These symbols are not concepts or things to be analysed by the mind but experiences that you must have personally:

The true nature of consciousness is certainly empty and without a base; it is not concrete, like empty space. Contemplate your own consciousness to understand if this is really so.

This is not the emptiness of the nihilist view, in fact spontaneous knowledge is certainly radiant from the very beginning; it is self-arising and self-resplendent like the heart of the sun. Contemplate your own consciousness to understand if this is really so.

Awareness is certainly unceasing from the very beginning; it is like the main current of a river that flows continuously. Contemplate your own consciousness to understand if this is really so.

Commentary

> Mental fluctuations certainly cannot be grasped; they are movements without solidity like a breeze in the sky. Contemplate your own consciousness to understand if this is really so.
>
> All phenomena, whatever they are, are certainly our own manifestations; whatever appears is like our reflection in a mirror. Contemplate your own consciousness to understand if this is really so.
>
> All [mental] images certainly dissolve spontaneously; they arise by themselves and dissolve by themselves like clouds in the sky. Contemplate your own consciousness to understand if this is really so.

In spite of this there are still some that cannot understand. But who is the one that has doubts, that thinks, that observes, that meditates, that seeks, that acts, that strives, that does not understand? Who is it that says, "It is I?" Has it got form or colour? Seeking it this way you will not find it, yet, do you not feel yourself?

Both in the absence of thoughts and in their presence, in a pleasant sensation and an unpleasant one, walking or staying still, talking or remaining silent, in whatever circumstance, is there still the feeling of oneself?

Before, during and after any operation by the mind and by the body the feeling of consciousness is always present; however most people are not aware of it because they are living as if in a dream, completely distracted.

Distraction gives rise to lack of self-control in thoughts, words and deeds; and behaviour that is out of harmony causes suffering to oneself and to others. Nevertheless, just as any reflection can appear in a limpid mirror, so, enlightened consciousness remains unaltered from the very beginning, making both the illusory dream and the subsequent awakening possible:

26. I, enlightened consciousness, the sovereign creator of all, am the mirror in which you observe all reality; everything appears in it clearly, yet devoid of a separate existence, therefore. . . .

Therefore, all the philosophies and practices of religions converge in the revelation and contemplation of the true nature of our consciousness:

> *There is nothing but consciousness; apart from this there is no view from which to observe. There is nothing but consciousness; apart from this there is no meditation to practise. There is nothing but consciousness; apart from this there is no conduct to apply. There is nothing but consciousness; apart from this there is no commitment to keep. There is nothing but consciousness; apart from this there is no goal to realize.*

The Tantra too confirms the same principle:

27. There is nothing besides me, so it is certain that there is no view on which to meditate. There is no [commitment] to keep besides me, so it is certain that there is no commitment to keep. There is nothing to seek besides me, so it is certain that there is no deed of power to seek. There is no other level besides me, so it is certain that there are no levels [to attain] by training.

From the very beginning there is no obscuration in me, so it is certain that I am spontaneous knowledge. I am the true nature of unborn reality, so it is certain that I am also subtle reality. There is nothing to travel besides me, so it is certain that there is no path to travel. The Buddhas, common beings and all reality come forth from me, the enlightened matrix, so it is certain that [in me] from the very beginning there is no duality.

As [I am] spontaneous knowledge free of doubts it is certain that I am also the great revelation that sweeps away doubts. As there is nothing besides me it is certain that I, the creator of all, am all. Not knowing me is the essence of obstacles. By seeking something besides me, deviations arise.

Commentary

For those who still have doubts, there is a further instruction on the symbol of celestial space:

> *Contemplate often, contemplate your own consciousness. Observing outwards, out in celestial space, there is no place towards which consciousness moves. Observing inwards, here inside your own consciousness, there is no one who moves with thought. Hence, your own consciousness is luminously resplendent without sparkling.*
>
> *The clear light of self-awareness is empty, [so] it is the reality body; like the sun arising in a bright cloudless sky, it knows everything clearly but without any concepts. There is a great difference between understanding it and not understanding it.*

Outer and inner space are not really separate, yet most people live as if they were. This happens because people are accustomed to projecting their mental images both onto themselves and onto objects, whereby they end up believing in the self and the other made up and separated illusorily by those images. However, when we relax without getting distracted the mental images dissolve naturally into all-supporting consciousness. In this state of naked awareness there is no separation between outer and inner space:

> 28. Oh! This state of being that is governed by awareness, creator of all, is ineffable and unimaginable; as memories have been stilled, it is free of lucubration; like the sky, it is omnipresent and boundless.

By letting your deceptive projections dissolve in a natural way, like clouds in the sky, the sun of consciousness shines, illuminating boundless space. When this happens even for just a moment, self-awareness is no more associated with any mental image, so it is impossible to identify it, saying: "It is this"; yet everything can be known as it is.

> *Incredible! This clear light, unborn from the very beginning and natural, is awareness, the young child without father or mother. Not produced by anybody, it is spontaneous knowledge. Not having experienced birth, it does not die.*

Incredible! Although it shines directly, there is no observer. Even though one wanders in transmigration, it does not become something bad. Even though one attains liberation, it does not become something good.

Incredible! Although it exists everywhere, it is not understood. [Even though it is] the goal, people neglect it, wishing for another goal. Even though it is oneself, people seek it elsewhere.

Naked awareness is not a theory to study; it does not depend on a concrete or conceptual support upon which to concentrate, or on a rule of conduct to apply by training in specific activities. Nor it is the result of a long quest:

Marvellous!

This awareness of the present moment, indeterminable and clear, is indeed the utmost peak of all views.

Without an image as support, omnipresent, not bound by the mind, it is indeed the utmost peak of all meditations.

This unaltered state of relaxation without any attachment is indeed the utmost peak of all conducts.

This realization, innate from the very beginning and not sought at all, is indeed the utmost peak of all goals.

If there is effort, it means that you are still trying to scale the mountain or climb the tree; however, the utmost peak transcends the concept of something to achieve:

29. It is said that I, enlightened consciousness, sovereign creator of all, am the utmost peak of all the teachings. The various systems of ethical rules, of instructions, of philosophical studies and of Tantras, the [texts of] one hundred thousand [verses], the secret creation [process] and the secret completion [process], etc., which have been taught by the three bodies of the masters that have come forth from me, imply effort. All try in this way to reach me, I who am beyond

Commentary

effort, but so doing they will not see me. That is why I am said to be the utmost peak of all the teachings.

The same principle can be expressed in another way by the example of the threads and nails used to mark the cross that divides the space in a sacred circle. The knowledge of awareness is the actual real meaning of the threads and nails.

I will explain the four great straight threads.

The great thread of right view is this limpid feeling of the present moment; it is called "thread" because it is clear and does not allow errors.

The great thread of right meditation is this limpid feeling of the present moment; it is called "thread" because it is clear and does not allow errors.

The great thread of right conduct is this limpid feeling of the present moment; it is called "thread" because it is clear and does not allow errors.

The great thread of the right goal is this limpid feeling of the present moment; it is called "thread" because it is clear and does not allow errors.

I will explain the four great firm nails.

The great nail of the unchanging view is just this limpid feeling of the present moment; it is called "nail" because it is stable in the three times.

The great nail of unchanging meditation is just this limpid feeling of the present moment; it is called "nail" because it is stable in the three times.

The great nail of unchanging conduct is just this limpid feeling of the present moment; it is called "nail" because it is stable in the three times.

> *The great nail of the unchanging goal is just this limpid feeling of the present moment; it is called "nail" because it is stable in the three times.*

When you understand that all reality exists from the very beginning in the single point of enlightened consciousness, then there is no need to draw the circle of the deities or to imagine their gradual or instantaneous radiation from the central point and subsequent reabsorption into it.

The views, meditations, conducts and goals that imply effort and alteration are mutable because they change according to personal inclinations, and can lead one astray like the many branches of a tree. It is true that also in this teaching the instructions are diversified, nevertheless they all converge on a single point, which is unborn, has not become, is uncreated and uncompounded:

30. O Great Being, listen! As all reality has the nature of a great point, it is free of unfolding and contracting, it is not subject to birth or to cessation, it is eternally what is. This matrix free of mental images exists from the very beginning like space, so it is beyond concept and verbal expression.

A teaching like this is unchanging and free of errors because it does not concern the past or the future and does not require altering the present; it only consists in naked awareness here and now. . . .

RN: What is your experience?

GB: My mind continues creating images, moreover when I am present to myself I have the experience of being so, as if a part of me were saying: "This is it." Does this mean that I am not yet in the true state of naked awareness? But you said that simply feeling myself here and now is already that state. I don't understand.

RN: You should not have any doubts about the fact that the essence of your actual awareness is the same as awareness completely released from mental images. Even if during the day the sky is cloudy, the natural light that illuminates the world is the same as the sun that shines beyond the clouds, just as the sky is the same both sides of the clouds.

So, don't worry about mental images; worrying itself is another conditioning image and in any case the light and dark clouds too have a role in the natural order of things. Let them come and go naturally. The simple feeling of being present, the natural thought of "I" or "me" is the spontaneous knowledge of self-awareness. . . .

Still, learn not to get your mind stuck even in that feeling. Stop commenting on all your states of consciousness and relax in the natural state.

Be! When you are instead of trying to be, what need is there to say: "This is it"? You are that by nature, by the very fact of existing, without needing to seek it, conceptualise it or to establish it in an experience.

* * *

Here is the instruction that enables you to abide in the unity of the three times.

Not attending to the past, leave any considerations about what has passed; not anticipating the future, cut the bonds of mental associations; not grasping the present, remain in the condition of space.

As there is nothing on which to meditate, do not meditate on anything, and as there is no reason to get distracted, rely on undistracted presence. Without meditating, without getting distracted, simply observe.

Self-awareness, feeling oneself that arises limpidly and shines by its own light, is enlightened consciousness. There is nothing on which to meditate, in fact it is beyond the knowable; there is no distraction, in fact it is clear by nature. Empty phenomena resolve themselves spontaneously, and empty clarity is the reality body.

Basically, the third introduction to awareness makes use of the symbol of space. In fact, empty space is not something that can be grasped either with the body or with the mind, so it has always been considered the most significant symbol of the original state:

31. Thus, just as all reality exists in space, so Buddhas, common beings and various things abide in the supreme universal state of enlightened consciousness.

In this case too, it is not a matter of reflecting on the symbol with your mind or of focusing on space in front of you. It is enough for you to remain relaxed and aware but with your attention open, as spacious as the sky. Innumerable objects can be present outside, many thoughts can arise within; whatever appears in your field of consciousness, remain natural, relaxed yet aware. And what if you do get distracted? Well, sooner or later you notice you have become distracted, don't you? This pure self-remembering is the very presence of awareness:

32. Thus, the secret instruction on the heart of non-meditation is to maintain the state of presence without getting distracted.

When there is the presence of awareness, everything becomes clear naturally. Striving to obtain enlightenment by altering body, voice and mind is like wanting to settle water by shaking the vessel containing it:

33. The unaltered natural state is the true nature of all reality; beyond the true nature of reality there is no state of enlightenment. "Buddha" is just a name, the "true nature of reality" is nothing but one's own consciousness; the unaltered state of one's own consciousness is called the "reality body." From the very beginning the unaltered state is unborn, so what is unborn does not need effort and striving. The state of non-action is not realized by effort and striving.

Spontaneous self-knowledge, pure and luminous by nature, is called "Diamond Being." In fact, enlightenment is awakening to what we really are, here and now, in every moment and in any place. Padmasambhava affirms it with these words:

Commentary

As it is the manifestation of enlightenment not realized by means of a path it is the vision of Diamond Being in this very moment.

When we don't understand this principle we elaborate an image of what we would like to become and contrive a path to achieve it by gradually correcting what we believe ourselves to be. Therefore, the Tantra teaches thus:

34. There are no gradual paths to achieve me; as spontaneous knowledge is complete in one moment it is achieved by abiding in the natural state without travelling [a path].

Now let us remain in silence. . . .

RN: Is everything clear?

GB: I don't understand. It seems to me that presence, as I experience it, is still a mental state veiled by images.

RN: When you think that, you are judging, so you have already altered what is. Leave your judgements to dissolve in the luminous, indeterminable space of your natural state as it is in the present moment.

GB: But presence entails the recognition of distraction, and isn't this itself already judgement?

RN: Presence serves to bring you back to yourself, like when you notice that you are dreaming; but if you struggle to maintain presence by fixing on it this means you are trying to climb the tree and thus are no longer the tree.

If you remain in your natural state, also letting the concept of presence vanish, then the concept of distraction too will disappear. Then you will be aware without knowing that you are.

* * *

Here is the teaching on the definitive consumption.

Although there are countless conflicting views, in spontaneous knowledge, in the true nature of self-aware consciousness, there is no duality of observer and observed.

Do not have a point of view, [rather] seek the observer. When, seeking the observer, you do not find the observer, then the view has been consumed; right here you also achieve the final view.

There is no point of view from which to observe; however, without falling into nihilist indifference, limpid feeling oneself in the present moment is the view of the great understanding. Here there is no duality of understanding and not understanding.

Although there are countless conflicting meditations, in the omnipresent ordinary feeling of self-awareness there is no duality of meditation and meditator.

Do not meditate, [rather] seek the meditator. When, seeking the meditator, you do not find the meditator, then meditation has been consumed; right here you also achieve the final meditation.

There is no meditation to engage; however, without letting yourself be overcome by the various forms of torpor and agitation, clear unaltered feeling of the present moment is contemplation of the even and uncontrived state. Here there is no dualism of calm and agitation.

Although there are countless conflicting conducts, in the single point of self-aware knowledge there is no duality of conduct and one who applies it.

Do not practise a conduct, [rather] seek the one who is practising it. When, seeking the one who is practising it, you do not find its practitioner, then the conduct has been consumed; right here you also achieve the final conduct.

There is no conduct to apply; however, without letting yourself be conditioned by the illusion of latent tendencies, the feeling of the present moment, unaltered and self-resplendent, in which there is nothing to correct, modify, obtain or give up, is itself absolutely pure conduct. Here there is no duality of pure and impure.

Although there are countless conflicting goals, in the true nature of self-aware consciousness the three bodies [of the Buddhas] are an innate realization. Here there is no duality of realization and the one who realizes.

Do not seek to realize the goal, [rather] seek just the one who realizes it. When, seeking the one who realizes it, you do not find him or her, then the goal has been consumed; right here you also achieve the final goal.

There is no goal to realize; however, without letting yourself be conditioned by rejection and obtainment, by hope and fear, understand that the self-replendent feeling of the present moment is innate realization, because here, within oneself, the three bodies are fully manifest; precisely this is the goal of original enlightenment.

The fourth introduction to awareness is concerned mainly with the ultimate meaning of the view, meditation, conduct and goal. This principle is important not only for Buddhists but also for anybody who has a faith or professes a religion in order for spirituality not to degenerate into its opposite. Unfortunately, this has already taken place and continues to do so the moment that followers of individual doctrines claim that they are the defenders or sole messengers of the only truth. However, the definitive and everlasting teaching is beyond the limited and transitory forms represented by any religion.

There is nothing existing in time and space that lies outside the process of continuous becoming through the consumption of old forms and the assumption of new ones. Even the personality changes, fortunately; yet, people tend to block this process by getting stuck in a particular world-view and by taking up rigid behaviour. It is in consequence of this that, in the field of spirituality too, institutions, associations, groups and centres arise, each with its own specific theories and practices and each claiming to be the sole holder of the truth. But how can the single truth still be bound to names, speculations, rites, meditations, rules and particular experiences?

When my master realized the complete extinction of the dualistic mind, his life changed radically. In order to avoid problems with the authorities, as he was certain they would not understand, he left his monastery and retreated to a hermitage, where only a few disciples could find him. I too went to visit him in that wild place. At that time I had not yet received this teaching so I was surprised by his behaviour, but I was not outraged because my faith in him was absolute. I noticed my master did not do any more formal practice and did not even bestow the initiations to which we were accustomed. He continued to give teachings of various kinds, according to his disciples' capacities, however in a style that was much simpler than before. Moreover, on specific occasions he also performed rituals for his disciples but his actions were new and I did not know their meaning.

One fine day I decided to ask the master what his spiritual practice was. He remained silent, perfectly still, staring into my eyes. Under the influence of his silence, I too became silent and entered, for a moment, into a limpid, non-conceptual state. After a while, I heard the master say that that was the direct transmission of the sacred wordless revelation, the teaching beyond scriptures and symbols.

The master explained that, when dualistic perception ceases completely, the mind cannot fall back on itself, no act of mental reflection is possible and the faculty of imagination stops operating. However, the physical senses and the intellect function perfectly yet effortlessly and activities are performed spontaneously, without any personal intention. Then he recited this passage from the revelation to corroborate what he had just told me:

35. O king of knowledge, Diamond Being, listen! The teaching of
   [what is known as] the definitive doctrine on the absolute

[reality] is not something the king of knowledge can know and explain. It is not something one can establish on nor is it an object of the imagination. It cannot be conceptualized, by nature it is beyond judgements. It cannot be meditated on through concentration, it is not bound by the mind. Desire is absent, so it is not a fruit to be reaped.

Therefore, whoever abides in reality as it is without judging achieves enlightenment without having travelled a path. He or she discovers spontaneous knowledge without having trained their awareness. Deeds of power are accomplished naturally without endeavour. One is pure by nature without having to keep commitments.

In reality as it is, objects and the senses are clear, Buddhas and common beings are not perceived as different, and there is the feeling that everything is one in reality as it is. There is neither unity nor plurality in reality as it is. Regarding the matrix that was never born, how can one express an opinion?

My master told me that those words were addressed expressly to me; then he added that from that moment, instead of studying, meditating, complying with rules and seeking the results of practice, I should observe myself and seek who I was. It was at that moment that my religion appeared to me as merely an assemblage of mental images with which I had illusorily identified myself.

Then the master transmitted to me Padmasambhava's instructions on the definitive consumption of view, meditation, conduct and goal. Oh, I followed them, for sure! But I ended up transforming them into a new creed and another method, believing that the institutions, theories and practices of my old religion were completely useless, if not even harmful. I spoke of this to my master. In order to help me understand the real meaning of Dzogchen, he explained that all the aspects of reality, also those of the religion I no longer agreed with, were nothing but expressions of the single enlightened consciousness and, thus, parts of the indivisible whole. Then he gave me this advice:

"If you believe there are contradictions in the explanations you have received, it is because you separate absolute and relative, wisdom and means. Never forget that the spontaneous knowledge realized by the sage is not an arid abstraction, it actually manifests in daily life as true love towards all beings and forms of life. Sages are free of the illusion of duality and yet they also know how to give the right toys to children. Nevertheless, they never try at any cost either to create or destroy anything because they live conjoined with enlightened consciousness that is the true maker of all. Sages remain effortlessly in the natural state, letting forms appear and disappear spontaneously, in accord with the natural order of things. When children grow up, they leave behind their old games in a natural way, like a snake shedding its skin or a tree its leaves. Only the person who does not know how to merge wisdom and means struggles vehemently to modify reality and ends up causing only suffering."

RN: Have you understood?

GB: I think so, but I do have one question: Is the state of consciousness where there is no longer the one that has a view, that meditates, that engages in a conduct, that seeks the goal, etc., the naked awareness free of mental images?

RN: It is the state of being in which the sense of separation between the self and the world ceases, but you are already experiencing that state albeit in an analogous way.

GB: I don't understand how.

RN: By living in your natural state, not in the one you would like to realize but instead just what you are in the present moment. Let your feeling express itself freely without any longer hoping for liberation or fearing transmigration.

GB: Then, what is the point of the teaching on a state of consciousness free of mental images?

RN: Some people understand this instruction the moment they receive it because they are ready and enter that state immediately.

GB: So I am not ready yet.

RN: You are still discriminating. Do not judge yourself. Be in the present. Be natural, and everything that must be shall be, just as everything already is.

GB: What does that mean, that everything already is?

RN: It means that, in reality, there is already awakening but you don't think so because you compare yourself with somebody else, you think that you have to experience it in a different way and so you aren't present in the present. Comparison, as you live it, entails a negative evaluation and, thus, alteration. When you are really aware in the present you don't alter anything because you don't judge yourself, you simply are.

GB: What you said about love made me think that we should also develop love for ourselves, for example when, comparing ourselves with great teachers, we consider ourselves inept or succumb to the frustration of imperfection.

RN: Right! Stop comparing yourself with anybody and love yourself; in this way you will be able to understand others' needs and will know how to help when asked. Be yourself genuinely and respect others, letting them really be themselves. This is the way to become masters of self-liberation.

* * *

Now there are some instructions addressed particularly to those who are not able to understand the preceding teachings:

> *This awareness, unbound by the eight limits of permanence and cessation [etc.], is called the "middle way" inasmuch as it does not fall into those extremes. It is called "awareness" because presence is unceasing. It is given the name "essence of the realized beings" because it is emptiness that has the nature of awareness.*

When there is this understanding one transcends all the knowable, thus it is also called "transcendent knowledge." Beyond the mind, from the very beginning it is not bound by the extremes of conclusions, so it is given the name "great seal."

Due to the difference between understanding it and not understanding it, it becomes the basis of all the happiness and suffering of liberation and transmigration so that it is called "universal base." Just this ordinary, common, everyday feeling, clear and limpid, is given the name "ordinary feeling."

However many pleasant names and beautiful definitions there may be, really whoever aspires to something more, to something different from this feeling of the present moment, is like someone who follows the footsteps of an elephant in spite of having already found it. Even if he follows [its footsteps] in the numerous worlds, he will never find [the elephant]; in the same way, aside from consciousness enlightenment can never be found.

Not having understood it, one seeks consciousness outside; however, how can one find oneself by seeking oneself in what is other than oneself? It is like an idiot giving up his own identity in order to mimic many people and, subsequently, no longer recognizing himself, looking for himself elsewhere and confusing himself with someone else.

Most seek Buddha-nature outside themselves, in a master or another higher being they consider divine, and through worshipping these entities they hope to obtain not only ordinary powers but also ultimate liberation.[11] Yet the Tantra states:

36. Those who consider the state of enlightenment as an entity will not find it, as they disregard the true nature of reality; so do not look at the Buddha but rather understand your own consciousness free of action.

---

11. Ordinary powers are various forms of magical dominion over matter.

Commentary

Our contemporary societies, both in the East and the West, are very far from applying this truth. Yet there was a time when people did not try to accumulate knowledge through study, did not strive to develop abilities and powers, did not impose rules of conduct on themselves and did not pursue goals driven by hope and fear, because they knew how to live in the natural way, relying solely on their spontaneous knowledge as the source of all true learning and capacity.

Then along came some people who started seeking knowledge, powers, certainty and security outside themselves. That was when the original harmony was broken and the affliction of effort spread, contaminating the majority, and in the world there appeared discrimination, inequality, conflict and the evils that still endure to this day. Why did all this come about and how can we return to our original condition?

By observing yourself it is not difficult to discern that the root of the current situation of confusion and suffering is a kind of ignorance or misunderstanding characterized by distraction. In fact, what often happens when we experience sensations, emotions, thoughts and fantasies is that we forget what we really are and end up believing we are what we are experiencing; from this there arise conditioning, dependence, disharmony, lack of self-control and suffering.

Not seeing the real condition of things, we do not understand that phenomena are consciousness, so we deviate into transmigration. Not understanding that enlightenment is our own consciousness, liberation is obscured.

Transmigration and liberation are no more different from each other than understanding and not understanding are in their single instant; we are deluded when we see them as other than our own consciousness.

Illusion and disillusion are of one essence; in a being there are not two threads of consciousness, so illusion dissolves when we leave consciousness itself in its own unaltered natural state.

The true nature of our consciousness is unconditioned, pure and luminous from the very beginning; however, when we do not recognize it and get distracted, this is like dreaming, convinced that the dream images really exist in a way that is concrete and independent of us. Accomplishing enlightenment is like recognising that we are dreaming, rediscovering self-awareness and reawakening. Until we understand this truth then the very search for enlightenment itself perpetuates the illusion of transmigration. Thus, transmigration and liberation are nothing but ignorance and understanding of our true nature. In an instant we fall asleep, in an instant we reawaken. Who is asleep, and who is awake?

Illusion and disillusion are like the pearls threaded on the single thread of a necklace. Whoever understands the nature of that single thread knows the true, essential, mutual and ultimate meaning of all the sacred texts.[12] In order to recognize this elementary truth it is enough to remain in the natural state. Water cannot regain its natural limpidity as long as we continue forcefully shaking the vessel that contains it.

The preceding indication is enough for some people, whereas others need further explanations. In this case it might be useful to observe the sensations, emotions and thoughts that follow one another in the arena of our consciousness:

When not aware of the fact that illusion itself is consciousness, not understanding at all the true nature of reality, you should observe by yourself and within yourself that which arises spontaneously.

While observing this display you must pay attention to the place where inner phenomena arise, manifest and, then, disappear:

At the beginning, whence do these phenomena arise? Then, where do they abide? Finally, where do they vanish? Observe them as if

---

12. "Thread" and "text" render one Tibetan word *rgyud* (Skr. *tantra*). The Tibetan word *mdo* (Skr. *sūtra*), another kind of sacred text, has the same meaning.

Commentary

> they were crows on a boat [in the middle of the sea]; they fly off from the boat but they have no other place to alight. In the same way, phenomena arise from consciousness and dissolve in it.

If you are not distracted, you recognize that that single mysterious place is only your own consciousness. The state of naked awareness precedes concepts and emotions because it is their original base, like the sky where clouds naturally appear and dissolve:

> The true nature of consciousness, empty clarity that feels everything and is aware of everything, is like space in which clarity and emptiness are inseparable from the beginning. Ascertaining clearly and directly that it is spontaneous knowledge, this itself is the real condition. Here is the proof: you understand that all phenomena are consciousness and that the nature of consciousness, being clear awareness, is like space.

> Although the example of space is used to point out the real condition, it is only a symbol that indicates it partially. The nature of consciousness is endowed with awareness, an emptiness that is utterly clear; space is unaware, an emptiness devoid of matter. This is the reason why the nature of consciousness cannot really be indicated by [the example of] space. Remain in the condition [of space] without getting distracted.

Those inclined to use the rational mind could try to understand this teaching by means of logic and erroneously conclude that their original nature is empty like immaterial space, however space is only a symbol. Its meaning is the real natural state of consciousness.

> One cannot demonstrate the real existence of any of the diverse phenomena as they appear conventionally; in fact they disappear.

If you are unable to remain in your natural state like in space, without clinging to anything or judging anything and instead soon let yourself get conditioned by sensations, then you must observe the nature of phenomena.

Do not analyse phenomena, rather observe them without getting distracted. If you try to observe phenomena in this way, you will discover that what you believed was the object disappears and, in its place, there is reality free of mental images.

Observe both the person you love best and the one you hate most, the thing you find most precious or pleasant and the one you find most tawdry or unpleasant, and you will see they appear as such only by imagining them in that way.

> *To exemplify that, [consider] all reality, transmigration and liberation, to be only the manifestation of your own consciousness. When [your] state of consciousness changes the corresponding manifestation appears externally.*

In fact, things as they appear depend on our state of consciousness, on understanding or not understanding ourselves, comparable to the limpid or murky conditions of the same water.

> *Thus, everything is a manifestation of consciousness. The six kinds of common beings hold distinct views of phenomena; outside [Buddhism], the extremists hold the dualistic view of permanence and cessation; and the nine levels of vehicles hold distinct views.*

All beings see things differently, conditioned by their own inclinations, preferences and desires:

> *You see various things and various things are not the same; so, as you grasp the differences, you are beguiled by personal attachment. When you are aware that all phenomena are consciousness, even though the perception of phenomena arises, by not grasping [it] you are Buddha.*

When there is no longer attachment to a subjective image of reality, what happens is that that image dissolves, you are no longer conditioned by personal inclinations and you reawaken from the dream.

Commentary

> *It is not phenomena that beguile, it is grasping them that beguiles. Grasping dissolves by itself when you are aware that it is consciousness.*

Actually, it is not phenomena that condition you, it is personal attachment to phenomena. How, then, is it possible to liberate yourself from attachment? By understanding that it too does not exist independently of your consciousness. When you abide in the state of naked awareness, subjective images naturally dissolve together with attachment and all the positive qualities manifest spontaneously.

> *Whatever appears is a manifestation of consciousness. The material vision of the external world, too, is consciousness. What appears as the six kinds of common beings, too, is consciousness; the beatific vision of the deities in their worlds and of humans is consciousness, and the painful vision of the three lower worlds is consciousness.*

> *What appears as the five emotional poisons, that is, misunderstanding [and the other poisons], is consciousness and what appears as the awareness of spontaneous knowledge, too, is consciousness.*

> *What appears as the latent traces of transmigration [determined by] negative thoughts is consciousness and what appears as the heavens of liberation [determined by] positive thoughts is consciousness.*

> *What appears as the obstacles of demons and evil forces is consciousness and what appears benign, such as deities and realizations, is consciousness.*

> *What appears as various concepts is consciousness and what appears as the non-conceptual state of concentration, too, is consciousness.*

> *What appears as the colour that characterizes things is consciousness and what appears as simple and devoid of characteristics, too, is consciousness.*

What appears as free of the dichotomy of unity and multiplicity is consciousness and what appears as utterly indeterminable as regards existence and non-existence, too, is consciousness.

In conclusion, you must understand that just as a dream and subsequently reawakening from it are made possible by our own consciousness, so the whole process of transmigration and liberation is sustained by a single base which is enlightened consciousness, the true nature of one's consciousness. In fact, the Tantra is explicit:

37. I am the natural state of everything; there is nothing besides my natural state. The masters [manifesting through] the three bodies are my natural state; the Buddhas of the three times are my natural state; the bodhisattvas are my natural state; the [practitioners of the] four Yogas are my natural state. The three worlds, of desire, of form and without form, too are indicated as my natural state, creator of all. The five elements too are my natural state; the common beings of the six conditions of existence, too, are my natural state. All phenomena are my natural state; all existence is my natural state; the entirety of worlds and of those living in them is my natural state. There is nothing besides my natural state, so all reality is comprised in me, I that am the root of everything; there is nothing that is not comprised in me.

Someone might ask: "If one's true nature is enlightened consciousness, then why does ignorance, the misunderstanding of actual reality, arise? How is it possible that enlightened consciousness itself, the natural state that is unborn, uncreated, free of becoming, eternal, uncompounded and free of suffering, manifests as that which is born, created, becoming, transitory, compounded and subject to suffering?" This is Padmasambhava's answer:

There is no phenomenon that is not consciousness. Whatever phenomenon appears [by virtue of] the unhindered nature of consciousness, although it arises, is like a wave in relation to the ocean; as there is no duality it resolves itself in consciousness itself.

Commentary

This means that, as it is not hindered by anything, enlightened consciousness manifests freely in any way, thus, also as the illusory condition of transmigration. In fact, the freedom of enlightened consciousness is also expressed in its capacity to hide its true nature because, otherwise, the enlightened ones, their teachings, the disciples, times and places would not exist:

38. I, the creator of all, am a secret to everyone. To the masters who have come forth from me [through] the three bodies I will not reveal my threefold natural state, it will remain a secret to them. I will not reveal my natural state to the Buddhas of the three times who abide in me, it will remain a secret to them. I will not reveal my natural state to the whole assemblies [of disciples] that surround [the masters] and converge in me, it will remain a secret to them. I will not reveal my natural state to the common beings of the three worlds created by me, it will remain a secret to them.

If I did not keep my natural state secret and were to reveal it, the masters [that manifest through] the three bodies would not come forth from me. If they did not come forth from me, the three teachings,[13] the three vehicles and the three kinds of disciples would not gather. If these did not gather there would not be the Three Jewels, that is the Buddha, his doctrine and his community, and nobody could know supreme enlightenment.

If I did not keep secret my natural state and were to reveal it to the Buddhas of the three times who have come forth from me, there would be the defect of the lack of the masters [who manifest through] the three bodies. If I did not keep secret my natural state and were to reveal it to the assemblies of disciples that converge in me, there would not be the subdivision of vehicles [taught by the] three masters. If due to compassion I

---

13. 1) The teaching of the emanation body (*nirmāṇakāya*) comprises the lesser vehicle (*hīnayāna*) and the greater vehicle (*mahāyāna*); 2) the teaching of the fruition body (*saṁbhogakāya*) comprises the esoteric traditions of the first three kinds of Tantras (*kriyā, ubhaya/caryā, yoga*); (3) the teaching of the reality body (*dharmakāya*) includes the remaining Tantras (*mahāyoga, anuyoga, atiyoga*).

were to reveal my natural state to common beings of the three worlds created by me, there would be no places for the three masters' teachings. And if that were the case, who could say that the reality created by me, the creator of all, is utterly complete?

Those who live distracted, unaware of their true nature, experience illusion and suffering. However, through suffering, sooner or later beings are spurred to seek its cause, and once they have found it, they also wish to discover the way to eliminate it; consequently, one day wisdom of understanding will arise from emotion. What makes possible and supports this whole process is nothing other than enlightened consciousness. But how does it hide and reveal itself, manifesting freely as the conditions of transmigration and of liberation?

39. So through its essence, existence and grace the sovereign creator of all creates all reality. From its single great spontaneous knowledge there originate the five great natural wisdoms,[14] those of aversion, of desire, of obtuseness, of envy and of pride. From these five natural wisdoms there originate five great ornamental causes and the three great transient worlds [of desire, of form and without form] are created. Grouping together all the bodies that constitute these causes we have the five bodies called earth, water, fire, air and ether.

Consequently:

40. The path of complete emancipation is fivefold: the five paths of the five natural wisdoms, indicated as the paths of all the Buddhas of the three times, are desire, aversion, obtuseness, envy and pride.

If you remain in your natural state, aware without altering reality as it is, concepts, mental images and emotions appear

---

14. "Spontaneous knowledge" and "natural wisdom" translate a single Tibetan expression, *rang 'byung ye shes*, that, however, has two distinct meanings, according to the context: the former is single self-awareness while the latter is the understanding arising from the experience of the five emotions.

and disappear naturally as waves of the same spontaneous knowledge. When there is this non-dual awareness it is possible to learn from any experience without remaining bound by it. It is in this way that naturally, without any effort at all, the beautiful lotus blooms on the water surface untainted by the mud, opening to the sunlight and closing at night.

After my master had realized the complete and irreversible dissolution of the dualistic mind, I asked him who or what was the "sovereign creator of all?" This was his answer: "Once I thought that the 'sovereign creator of all' was only one's own mind; now that the illusion of my little self has dissolved I see I was mistaken. If you ask me who or what it is I can only answer that I do not know because here the knower and the known are the same reality as it is." Then he chanted this passage from the Tantra:

41. Such is reality as it is; I too, the creator of all, am reality as it is, and that which is created by me, too, is reality as it is. The six sense objects are created by me. The sensory and mental faculties are my awareness. The entirety of [sensory and mental] consciousness is my spontaneous knowledge. The five elements, that is, the five causes of every thing, too are reality as it is. The five natural wisdoms [of my] grace, the three worlds and the six kinds of common beings are of the nature of reality as it is.

This is why the Tantra asserts that enlightened consciousness reveals its natural state only to itself, that is, in the condition of extreme union, true *Atiyoga*:

42. So I, the sovereign creator of all, will reveal to myself my natural state that I manifest. I, the creator of all, have not bestowed the doctrine that reveals [my natural state] to the masters and to their retinues, as they all come forth from me. The extreme union is me, the creator of all, hence that is where my natural state has to be revealed.

Now there follows the final advice.

> *Even though names are given due to the free presence of what is to be named, whatever the name is [that indicates authentic reality],*

> *in truth there is nothing but single consciousness; moreover, it is without a base, without a root.*

Authentic reality is called in many ways according to cultures and traditions, however it is nothing other than the single consciousness without a cause; that is why it is necessary to go beyond its different labels in order to rediscover the single original principle.

> *There is no unilateral point of view. Do not hold a concrete view because [consciousness] cannot be determined at all; do not hold the view of emptiness because there is the splendour of clear awareness; do not hold a fragmentary view because clarity and emptiness are inseparable.*

It transcends any conceptual determination, nevertheless it manifests freely everywhere and in every way; that is why it is important not to get stuck on any idea or experience and always to remain open, merging together wisdom and means.

> *Although feeling oneself in the present moment is clear and limpid, you do not know who it is that makes it so. It is impersonal, yet it can be experienced directly.*

You must not confuse naked awareness with an image of your limited I, but do not think that your true nature cannot be experienced here and now.

> *All [beings] can liberate themselves by experiencing this state [of pure awareness]. In fact, its recognition happens without any difference regarding the capacity [of understanding], whether it is sharp or dull.*

It is not necessary to become scholars or to undergo who knows what discipline in order to recognise it; however, nor should you remain indifferent, continuing to live distractedly, claiming that you are already enlightened from the very beginning:

> *Even though sesame and milk are the causes of oil and butter, if sesame is not ground and milk not churned there will be neither*

Commentary

> oil nor butter. Actually, all beings are potential Buddhas, but if they do not experience [awareness of their own true nature] they do not get enlightened, whereas even a herdsman gets liberated by experiencing it.

What is called enlightenment, salvation or realization is a potentiality that has to be awakened through self-awareness, in every moment and every circumstance. Even a poor ignoramus can awaken in this way.

> Although one does not know how to explain it, it can be ascertained directly; it is like tasting sugar so that you no longer need someone else to explain its flavour.

This teaching is only a pointer, but by applying it you can understand its true meaning, and when this happens there is no longer any need to rely on someone else's explanations. Padmasambhava was a great scholar and practitioner of Buddhist doctrines, both common and esoteric, yet he was only able to understand their single essential and ultimate meaning when his master, Śrī Siṁha, transmitted to him the direct introduction to awareness. Padmasambhava immediately put it into practice without prattling about it to others, so that he accomplished deep inner certainty and independence from any outer authority, becoming a master himself.

> Even great scholars are subject to delusion if they do not have this understanding. You can become expert in the field of the nine vehicles but it is like recounting a tale about something far away that you have never seen; in this way you do not approach enlightenment at all.

Nowadays serious disciples are rare; most make notes of the teaching but do not experience it deeply, and they even insist on writing books. How presumptuous!

43. Everyone talks about the true nature of consciousness [saying it is] unborn and everyone discusses the meaning of the impersonal state, but nobody understands the unborn directly.

Until this understanding blossoms you continue living bound by the illusory net of duality, causing suffering to yourself and to others.

If you have this understanding, virtue and vice dissolve spontaneously; if it is lacking, then whatever action you perform, whether it is virtuous or not, you will not transcend transmigration in the upper or lower worlds.

In this case it is better to learn self-control, submitting to a suitable discipline. In fact, the Tantra says:

44. The master of the masters, the sovereign creator of all, has taught that as long as you remain on the path of mental images you have a dualistic view that distinguishes between observing and not observing [rules], in which case you should keep the main and the secondary [vows]. I, the sovereign creator of all, have always been reality as it is. In reality as it is there is no subject and object, so whoever understands phenomena in this way does not conceive observing or not observing [rules].

Therefore, Padmasambhava teaches:

As soon as you understand the knowledge of your empty and clear consciousness there is no longer any real positive or negative consequence of virtuous or vicious actions. Just as a river does not gush out of empty space, so virtue and vice do not objectively exist in emptiness.

The Tantra too states this clearly:

45. Since all phenomena as they appear are one in the unborn true nature of reality, the distinction between obscuration and absence of obscuration cannot be ascertained in the essence of consciousness, the unborn matrix.

O Diamond Being, contemplate well! Whoever wishes to remove obscuration and obtain absence of obscuration, when [all] is one in the unborn true nature of reality, contradicts the authentic meaning of the supreme matrix. [. . .] Whoever remains beyond concepts and judgements as in space abides

Commentary

in enlightened consciousness, where there is neither obscuration nor absence of obscuration.

So, whoever has understood this essential teaching on the "unborn" has no commitments to keep except that of awareness; this means just remaining present, effortlessly and without fixations, in the natural state of self-liberation beyond both hope and fear:

46. As the true nature of reality never changes in the three times, understand that my commitment, the sovereign creator of all, is not to be kept in the three times. Oh, just as all reality is one single thing in the consciousness that constitutes its root, so commitments are one alone in [the commitment of] not keeping [that constitutes] the root [commitment], namely the understanding of one's unborn consciousness.

Thus, to see directly self-awareness in its nakedness, this teaching on natural liberation through seeing nakedly is really profound, so right here is where you must examine what self-awareness is. Deeply sealed.

Marvellous! This introduction to awareness, natural liberation through seeing nakedly, is a brief and clear synthesis composed taking into account the sacred scriptures, the revealed messages, the teachings of the masters and personal experience, with the aspiration to benefit the worthy ones of the dark age, those of future generations. At this time [the text] cannot be propagated; let it be concealed as a precious treasure. In future let it be discovered by the person destined to do so. Samayā. Sealed, sealed, sealed.

This text on direct introduction to awareness, called "Natural Liberation through Seeing Nakedly," was composed by Padmasambhava, Abbot of Uḍḍiyāna. May [this teaching] not end until transmigration has been emptied.

In Tibet Padmasambhava transmitted the essential instructions of Śrī Siṁha and Garab Dorje, integrating them with others taken from sacred texts and using as a basis his own experience. Among the disciples who received them there were his consorts Mandāravā and Yeshe Tsogyal, who transcribed them accurately. Subsequently, the master and his two great disciples hid the text so that it could be rediscovered and transmitted intact at a future time propitious for its promulgation. This happened when Karma Lingpa brought it to light on Mount Gampodar[15] and it continues to happen when someone rediscovers the true nature of consciousness.

At present, mankind is traversing a particular phase of a cosmic cycle. This temporary phase is dark because most people are no longer aware of their union with the Great Self so that tension, conflicts and suffering prevail everywhere. However even in the darkness of people's confused and afflicted mind the clear light of consciousness is shining. Whoever awakens to clear awareness of her or his true nature knows that the darkness is no more real than a hallucination.

RN: Do you still have questions?

GB: Yes. When I look for the place where thoughts arise, manifest and disappear I always find the feeling of existing as I. Instead, if I have understood you correctly, I should not find anything on which my mind can get stuck.

RN: This feeling itself is already the state of awareness, however for many people it is like the light of the sun behind thick dark clouds. When all the clouds disperse, the feeling of being, that is the thought "I," seems to dissolve completely. In actual fact, it is the illusion of being separate that dissolves, while the feeling oneself, which is unceasing, does not really dissolve but, instead, manifests as it has been from the very beginning: the "I am" of Kunje Gyalpo.

Don't worry about the clouds and don't even concentrate on the light, rather *be* the light that you already are without separating anything.

---

15. This mountain is situated in central Tibet. The rediscovery took place in the XIV century.

Commentary

GB: What do you mean by "not separating?"

RN: When you understand that all is one there is no longer transmigration or liberation, but this is already possible now because the light of the sun shines both in the space beyond the clouds and in the space this side of the clouds. The two spaces are one. You are that single space, just as you are that single light.

GB: Is that why Padmasambhava says that there is no real positive or negative consequence of actions?

RN: Certainly! The Primordial Buddha does not discriminate, does not separate, does not judge anything because he is spacious love that sustains and embraces all of life. That is why he is called Universal Goodness. As long as you separate cause and effect, you cannot be a master of *Atiyoga*.

GB: I know some *Atiyoga* teachings belonging to the three series of consciousness, of space and of advice that, according to your explanation, seem to me to pertain still to a path of cause and effect. Is that not a contradiction?

RN: According to the *Kunje Gyalpo* Tantra there are different categories of *Atiyoga* teachings.[16] The three series, of consciousness (*sems sde*), of space (*klong sde*) and of advice (*man ngag sde*), also prescribe methods based on the principles of cause and effect because they emphasise, respectively, the *atiyoga* phases of *sattvayoga*, of *mahāyoga* and of *anuyoga*.

The master Namkhai Norbu Rinpoche has transmitted to you the main methods of the three series and also the initiation to *Ati* beyond cause and effect, but have you realized its true meaning? In any case if you proceed in your quest with humility, I believe that in future you will have the opportunity

---

16. In Chapter 8 of the Tantra there is an explanation of the four paths of *yoga*: *sattvayoga*, *mahāyoga*, *anuyoga* and *atiyoga*. Each consists in four main phases called by the same names as the four *yogas*, therefore the fourth phase of each path is *atiyoga*.

to meet someone who will help you achieve a better understanding of those teachings in relation to the four paths of *yoga*. When you are ready to understand, the meeting will take place.

GB: But I have learnt that the *Kunje Gyalpo* Tantra is the fundamental text of the "consciousness series."

RN: That's right, however the "consciousness series" subsumes various groups of teachings. The *Kunje Gyalpo* Tantra stresses the *sattvayoga* phase of the *Atiyoga* path which discloses the original nature of consciousness. Whoever understands it is the supreme *sattva*, Diamond Being.

GB: I don't understand.

RN: Don't get lost in scholarly disquisition. There is only one thing that you need to know; knowing that, you can know everything: you are Kunje Gyalpo! You fail to accept this truth because you persist in separating the impure vision of ignorance from the pure vision of knowledge, but they are one single thing.

Consciousness, whether you consider it enlightened or not enlightened, is nothing but thought. Everything that happens to us, every thing that we perceive, is the natural manifestation of thought that is in us.

When you are distracted you can stumble. When you are aware you can walk without falling. Why are you distracted? Because you wanted to be distracted in order to manifest the wisdom of what it means to be distracted.

You can use the creative power of thought to manifest anything, but any manifestation is nothing but the free expression of the original thought, the splendour of spontaneous knowledge, the grace of enlightened consciousness. The original thought is the base that enables all of reality to be what it is because it is the totality of what is. So what is the sense of separating?

Commentary

In the sacred circle of this great city there is all of existence, the upper worlds and the lower worlds, the reality of liberation and that of transmigration. You have wandered its streets, old and new, you have allowed yourself to see and your heart has felt. But your judging mind continues to separate pure from impure. . . .

How difficult it is to communicate the secret of life!

What more can I say?

Listen. Imagine you are at the centre of a temple dedicated to the supreme deity. It is round, with a dome, and not even one ray of light comes in from outside. With both your hands you are holding a bright lamp, the only source of light in the temple. You look around and notice that it has no sacred images, there is just you and . . . countless mirrors of various shapes and sizes scattered everywhere, on the round wall, on the dome and on the floor. Now look at the mirrors and tell me what you see.

GB: In every mirror there is the image of me holding the lamp, but in different forms.

RN: Right! So stop separating yourself from other beings and from the Primordial Buddha. You are the "God of gods" (*lha'i lha*). . . . I am too, and like us so are other beings, because all is one. Oh! Isn't this revelation marvellous? There will come a day when all will be fully aware of it. That glorious day is not far. . . . In truth, it is already now.

Appendices

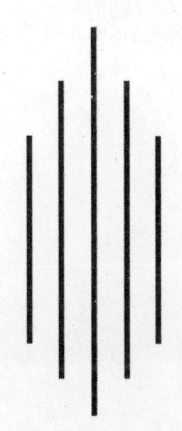

**Transliteration of
the
Tibetan Texts**

Appendix 1.

PHYAG RGYA CHEN PO'I MAN NGAG

/rdo rje[1] mkha' 'gro la phyag 'tshal lo//phyag rgya chen po bstan du med kyis kyang/[2]/dka' ba spyad[3] cing bla ma la gus pas[4]//sdug bsngal bzod ldan blo ldan nā ro pa//skal ldan khyod kyis[5] snying[6] la 'di ltar byos/[7]/dper na nam mkha' gang gis gang la brten//de bzhin[8] phyag rgya che la brten yul med//ma bcos gnyug ma'i ngang du glod[9] la zhog /bcings pa glod[10] na grol bar the tshom med//dper na nam mkha'i dkyil bltas mthong ba[11] 'gag par 'gyur//de bzhin sems kyis

---

1. B *dpal rdo rje*.
2. B omits this line.
3. A *spyod*.
4. B *pa*.
5. A *kyi*.
6. B *blo*.
7. B inserts /*phyag rgya chen po bstan du med kyis kyang*/.
8. B *rang sems*.
9. A *klod*.
10. A, B *klod*.
11. A *bar*.

sems la bltas byas na//rnam rtog tshogs 'gag bla med byang chub thob//dper na khug sna sprin rnams[12] nam mkha'i khams[13] su dengs//gar yang song ba med cing gang du'ang[14] gnas pa med//de bzhin sems las byung ba'i rtog tshogs kyang//rang sems mthong bas rtog pa'i rba rlabs dengs[15]//dper na nam mkha'i rang bzhin kha dog dbyibs las 'das//dkar nag dag gis gos shing 'gyur ba med//de bzhin rang sems snying po kha dog dbyibs las 'das//dge sdig dkar nag chos kyis gos mi 'gyur//dper na gsal dvangs[16] nyi ma'i snying po de//bskal pa stong gi mun pas bsgrib mi nus[17]//de bzhin rang sems snying po 'od gsal de//bskal pa'i 'khor bas bsgrib[18] par mi nus so//dper na nam mkha' stong par tha snyad rab btags[19] kyang//nam mkha' la ni 'di 'dra[20] brjod du med//de bzhin rang sems 'od gsal brjod gyur kyang//'di[21] 'drar grub ces tha snyad gdags gzhi med//de ltar sems kyi rang bzhin gdod nas nam mkha' 'dra//chos rnams ma lus[22] de ru ma 'dus med//lus kyi bya ba yongs thong[23] rnal ma[24] dal bar sdod//ngag gi smra brjod med de grag[25] stong brag cha 'dra//yid la ci yang mi bsam la bzla'i chos la ltos//lus la snying po med de

---

12. B *dper nas rlangs sprin ni.*
13. B *dbyings.*
14. B *gar yang.*
15. B *dvangs.*
16. B *dvang.*
17. B *sgrib mi 'gyur.*
18. B *sgrib.*
19. B *brtags.*
20. B *'drar.*
21. B *brjod pas 'dir.*
22. B *thams cad.*
23. B *thongs.*
24. B *'byor.*
25. A *brag.* B *grags.*

Phyag rgya chen po'i man ngag

smyug[26] ma'i sdong po 'dra//sems ni nam mkha'i dkyil ltar bsam pa'i yul las 'das//de yi ngang la btang bzhag med par glod[27] la zhog /sems la[28] gtad so med na phyag rgya chen po yin//de la goms shing 'dris na bla med byang chub thob// sngags su smra dang pha rol phyin pa dang//'dul ba mdo sde sde snod sna tshogs kyi[29] //rang rang gzhung dang grub pa'i mtha' yis ni//'od gsal phyag rgya chen po mthong mi 'gyur/ /zhe 'dod byung bas 'od gsal ma mthong bsgribs//rtog pa'i bsrung[30] sdom dam tshig don las nyams//yid la mi byed zhe 'dod kun dang bral//rang byung rang zhi chu yi rba rlabs[31] 'dra//mi gnas mi dmigs don las mi 'da' na//dam tshig mi 'da' mun pa'i sgron me yin//zhe 'dod kun bral mtha' la mi gnas na//sde snod chos rnams ma lus mthong bar 'gyur// don 'dir gzhol na 'khor ba'i btson las thar//don 'dir mnyam bzhag sdig sgrib thams cad bsreg[32] /bstan pa'i sgron me zhes su bshad pa yin//don 'dir mi mos skye bo blun po rnams// 'khor ba'i chu bos rtag tu khyer bar zad//[33] sdug bsngal mi bzod[34] blun po snying re rje//sdug bsngal[35] mi bzod[36] thar 'dod bla ma mkhas la brten[37]//byin rlabs snying la zhugs nas[38] rang sems grol bar[39] 'gyur//kye ho/ 'khor ba'i chos 'di don

---

26. B *pa smyugs*.
27. A *klod*.
28. B *pa*.
29. B *la sogs pa*.
30. B *srung*.
31. B *pa tra*.
32. B *sreg*.
33. B inserts *ngan song*.
34. A *zad*. B *bzad*.
35. B omits *sdug bsngal*.
36. B *bzad*.
37. B *bsten*.
38. B *na*.
39. B *par*.

med sdug bsngal rgyu//byas pa'i chos la snying po med pas don ldan snying po ltos//gzung 'dzin kun las 'das na lta ba'i rgyal po yin//yengs pa med na sgom[40] pa'i rgyal po yin//bya rtsol[41] med na spyod pa'i rgyal po yin//re dogs med na 'bras bu mngon du 'gyur//dmigs pa'i yul 'das sems kyi rang bzhin gsal//bgrod pa'i lam med sangs rgyas lam sna zin//bsgom[42] pa'i yul med[43] bla med byang chub thob//kye ma 'jig rten chos la legs rtogs dang//rtag mi thub ste rmi lam sgyu ma 'dra//rmi lam sgyu ma don la yod ma yin//des na skyo ba skyed[44] la 'jig rten bya ba thong[45]//'khor yul chags sdang 'brel pa kun chod la[46]//gcig pur nags 'dab[47] ri khrod dgon par sgoms[48]//bsgom du med pa'i ngang la gnas par gyis//thob med thob na phyag rgya chen po thob[49]//dper na ljon shing sdong po yal ga lo 'dab rgyas//rtsa ba gcig bcad yal ga khri 'bum skam//de bzhin sems kyi rtsa ba bcad pas[50] 'khor ba'i lo 'dab skam//dper na bskal pa stong du[51] bsags pa'i mun pa yang//sgron me gcig gis mun pa'i tshogs rnams sel//de bzhin rang sems 'od gsal skad cig gis//bskal par bsags pa'i ma rig sdig sgrib sel//kye ho/ blo yi chos kyis blo 'das don mi mthong//byas pa'i chos kyis byar med don mi rtogs//blo 'das byar med don de thob 'dod na//rang sems rtsa ba chod la[52] rig pa gcer bur zhog /rtog pa dri ma'i chu de dvangs

---

40. B *bsgom*.
41. B *btsal*.
42. A *goms*.
43. B inserts *goms na*.
44. A *bskyed*.
45. B *thongs*.
46. B *gcod nas*.
47. B *'dabs*.
48. B *gnas par bsgom*.
49. B *'thob*.
50. B *na*.
51. B *skal stong* instead of *bskal pa stong du*.
52. B *rtsad chod* instead of *rtsa ba chod la*.

Phyag rgya chen po'i man ngag

su chug /snang ba dgag sgrub ma byed[53] rang sar zhog / spang blang med pa'i[54] snang srid phyag rgya che[55] //kun gzhi skye ba med pas[56] bag chags sgrib g.yogs sangs//snyems[57] byed rtsis gdab mi bya skye med snying por zhog /snang ba rang[58] snang blo yi chos rnams zad du chug /mu mtha' yongs grol lta ba'i rgyal po mchog /mu med gting yangs[59] sgom pa'i rgyal po mchog /mtha' chod phyogs bral spyod pa'i rgyal po mchog /re med rang gnas[60] 'bras bu'i mchog yin no//las ni dang po gcong rong 'bab chu 'dra//bar du chu bo gaṅgā[61] dal zhing g.yo/ /tha ma chu rnams ma bu 'phrad[62] pa 'dra//blo dman skye bo[63] ngang la mi gnas na//rlung gi gnad bzung rig pa bcud la bor//lta[64] stangs sems 'dzin yan lag du ma yis/ /rig pa ngang la mi gnas bar[65] du gcun[66] //las kyi phyag rgya bsten na bde stong ye shes 'char//thabs dang shes rab byin brlabs[67] snyoms par 'jug /dal bar dbab cing bskyil bzlog drang[68] ba dang//gnas su bskyal la[69] lus la khyab par

---

53. B *mi byar*.
54. B *len med par*.
55. B *rgyar grol*.
56. B *par*.
57. B *snyem*.
58. B *rab*.
59. A *yongs*.
60. B *grol*.
61. A *gang gā*.
62. A *phrad*.
63. B *skyes bu'i*.
64. B *lte*.
65. B *par*.
66. B *gtsun*.
67. B *rlabs*.
68. B *drangs*.
69. B *dang*.

dgram[70] //de la chags zhen med na bde stong ye shes 'char//
tshe ring skra dkar med cing zla ltar rgyas par 'gyur//bkrag
mdangs gsal la stobs kyang seng ge 'dra//thun mong dngos
grub myur thob mchog la gzhol bar 'gyur//phyag rgya chen
po gnad kyi man ngag 'di//'gro ba skal ldan snying la gnas
par zhog /phyag rgya chen po lhun gyis grub pa dpal te lo pa
chen po'i zhal snga nas mdzad pa/ kha che'i paṇḍi ta mkhas
pa grub pa thob pa nā ro pas dka' ba bcu gnyis spyad pa'i
mthar chu bo gaṅgā'i[71] 'gram du te lo pas gsungs pa/ phyag
rgya chen po rdo rje'i tshig rkang nyi shu rtsa brgyad pa zhes
bya ba nā ro pa chen po'i zhal snga nas/ bod kyi lo tsā[72] ba
chen po sgra sgyur gyi rgyal po mar pa chos kyi blo gros kyis
byang pu la ha rir bsgyur cing zhus te gtan la phab pa'o//

---

70. B *bya*.
71. A *gang gā'i*.
72. A *lotstsha*.

Appendix 2.

DO HA MDZOD CES BYA BA/

dpal rdo rje sems dpa' la phyag 'tshal lo//rang rig mi 'gyur phyag rgya chen po la phyag 'tshal lo//phung po khams dang skye mched rnams//phyag rgya chen po'i rang bzhin las// ma lus der byung de ru thim//dngos dang dngos med spros dang bral//yid la byar med don ma 'tshol//thams cad brdzun pa'i rang bzhin la//thog ma spang zhing tha ma spang//gang zhig yid kyi spyod yul gyur na de//gnas lugs ma yin tshu rol btags pa ste//de nyid bla mas ma yin slob mas min//sems dang sems med nyid du ma rtogs par//du ma spangs pa'i[1] gcig nyid go bar gyis//gcig la zhen na'ang de nyid kho nas 'cing//ti[2] lo ngas ni ci yang bstan du med//gnas ni dben pa ma yin mi dben min//mig ni phye ba ma yin btsums pa min/ /sems ni bcos pa ma yin ma bcos min//gnyug ma yid la byar med shes par gyis//chos nyid spros dang bral ba la//nyams myong[3] dran rig glo bur 'di//brdzun par rtogs na ci dgar thong//phung 'tshengs thob shor ci yang med//'bad de dka'

---

1. *spang ba'i.*
2. *te.*
3. *myang.*

thub nags la ma brten cig /khrus dang gtsang sbras bde ba mi rnyed do//lha rnams mchod kyang thar pa thob mi 'gyur// blang dor med pa'i rgya yan shes par gyis//rang gi de nyid rig pa 'bras bu yin//rtogs thob dus gcig lam la ltos pa med// 'jig rten rmongs pas gzhan du 'tshol bar byed//re dogs ltos pa bcad nas bde ba yin//gang du sems kyi ngar 'dzin zhi ba na//gnyis 'dzin snang ba de ni rab tu zhi//mi bsam mi mno brtag dpyad mi bya zhing//mi sgom mi spyod re dogs mi bya bar//der 'dzin blo yi 'du byed rang sar grol//dang po'i chos nyid steng du de yis phebs//do ha mdzod ces bya ba rnal 'byor gyi dbang phyug ti[4] lo pas mdzad pa rdzogs so// rgya gar gyi mkhan po bai ro tsa nas rang 'gyur du bsgyur ba'o//

---

4. te.

Appendix 3.

:ZAB CHOS ZHI KHRO DGONGS PA RANG GROL LAS:

RIG PA NGO SPROD GCER MTHONG RANG GROL BZHUGS SO:[1]

rig pa rang gsal sku gsum lha la 'dud[2]: zab chos zhi khro dgongs pa rang grol las: rig pa ngo sprod gcer mthong rang grol bstan: 'di ltar rang gi rig pa ngo sprod kyis[3]: legs par dgongs shig[4] skal ldan rigs kyi bu: sa ma yā: rgya rgya rgya: e ma ho: 'khor 'das yongs la khyab[5] pa'i sems gcig po[6]: ye nas

---

1. A *zhes bya ba bzhugs sho.*
2. A *phyag 'tshal lo.*
3. B *sprad kyi.*
4. A *cig.*
5. B *khyabs.*
6. B *pu.*

rang nyid[7] yin yang[8] ngo ma shes: gsal rig[9] rgyun chad med kyang zhal ma mjal[10]: 'gag med cir yang 'char te ngos ma zin: 'di nyid rang ngo shes par bya ba'i phyir: dus gsum rgyal bas chos sgo brgyad khri dang: bzhi stong la sogs bsam gyis mi khyab pa: gsungs[11] pa thams cad 'di nyid rtogs pa[12] las: gzhan du ci yang rgyal bas gsungs pa med: gsung[13] rab nam mkha'i[14] mtha' mnyam dpag med kyang: don la rig pa ngo sprod tshig gsum mo: rgyal ba'i dgongs pa mngon sum ngo sprod 'di: sba sri[15] med par[16] mdzub btsugs[17] 'di ka yin[18]: kye ho: skal ldan bu dag tshur nyon dang: sems zhes zer[19] ba'i yongs grags[20] sgra bo che[21]: 'di nyid ma rtogs log rtogs phyogs rtogs dang: yang dag ji bzhin nyid du ma rtogs pas: grub mtha'i 'dod pa bsam gyis mi khyab 'byung: de yang so so'i skye bo tha mal pas: ma rtogs rang ngo rang gis ma shes pas: khams gsum rgyud drug[22] 'khyams shing sdug bsngal spyod: de yang rang sems 'di nyid ma

---

7. A *bzhin*.
8. B *kyang*.
9. A *rigs*.
10. B *'jal*.
11. B *gsung*.
12. B *phyir*.
13. A *gsungs*.
14. A *mkha'*.
15. A *snga phyi*. B *bag sgrib*, however according to Rangdröl Naljor (henceforth RN) this should be emended to *sba sri*.
16. B *pa*.
17. A *'jug tshul*. Omitted in B. RN *mdzub btsugs*.
18. B *rang yin no*.
19. B *bya*.
20. A *sgrags*.
21. A *sgra che'o*.
22. B *rgyun nag*.

Rig pa ngo sprod

rtogs skyon: phyi rol mu stegs log par rtogs pa ste[23]: rtag chad mtha' la[24] lhung bas phyin ci log:[25] nyan thos rang rgyal phyogs tsam bdag med par: rtogs par 'dod kyang ji bzhin nyid[26] ma rtogs: gzhan yang rang rang[27] gzhung dang grub mtha' yi[28]: 'dod pas bcings pas 'od gsal ma[29] mthong zhing[30]: nyan thos rang rgyal gzung 'dzin zhen[31] pas bsgribs: dbu ma bden gnyis mtha' la zhen[32] pas bsgribs: kri yog bsnyen sgrub[33] mtha' la zhen[34] pas bsgribs: ma hā a nu dbyings rig zhen[35] pas bsgribs: gnyis med don la gnyis su phye[36] bas gol: gnyis med gcig tu ma gyur sangs mi rgya: thams cad rang sems 'khor 'das dbyer med la: spang blang[37] 'dor len theg pas 'khor bar 'khyams: rang rig sku gsum rtsol med lhun grub la: 'di min[38] thag ring gzhan du bgrod[39] thabs kyis: sa lam rtsi[40] ba'i rmongs pas don la g.yel[41]: sangs

---

23. B *de*.
24. B *las*.
25. A omits these two lines. B inserts *de yang rang sems 'di nyid ma rtogs skyon:*.
26. A *'di*.
27. B *gzhan*.
28. A *yis*. B *yas*.
29. A *mi*.
30. B *bsgrib*.
31. B *gzhen*.
32. B *gzhen*.
33. A *grub*.
34. B *gzhen*.
35. B *gzhen*.
36. B *dbye*.
37. A *dang*.
38. B *ming*.
39. B *sgrod*.
40. B *brtsi*.
41. B *yal*.

rgyas dgongs pa blo las 'das pa la: dmigs gtad mtshan ma'i sgom bzlas byed pa 'khrul[42]:[43] de phyir bcas bcos[44] bya bral kun bskyur[45] la: 'di ltar rig pa gcer mthong rang grol du: bstan pas chos kun rang grol chen por rtogs[46]: de phyir rdzogs pa chen por kun kyang rdzogs: sa ma yā: rgya rgya rgya: e ma ho: sems zhes zer ba'i rig rig tur tur po: yod ni gcig kyang yod pa ma yin te: byung ni 'khor 'das bde sdug thams cad[47] byung: 'dod[48] ni theg pa bcu gcig ltar du 'dod: ming ni bsam gyis mi khyab so sor btags: la la dag[49] gis[50] sems nyid sems nyid zer: mu stegs la[51] las[52] bdag ces[53] ming du btags: nyan thos pas ni gang zag bdag med[54] zer: sems tsam pas ni sems zhes ming du btags: la las dbu ma zhes pa'i[55] ming du btags:[56] la las shes rab pha rol phyin pa zer: la las bde gshegs snying po'i[57] ming du btags: la las phyag rgya chen po'i[58] ming du btags: la las thig le nyag gcig ming du btags: la las chos kyi dbyings zhes ming du btags: la las

---

42. B *khrul*.
43. A omits these five lines.
44. A, B *byas chos*.
45. A *bcud*. B *skyur*.
46. B *bsgoms*.
47. A *sna tshogs*.
48. B *'don*.
49. B *la las bdag*.
50. A *ni*.
51. B *pa*.
52. A *la*.
53. A *zhes*.
54. A *gdam ngag gdam ngag* instead of *gang zag bdag med*.
55. B *pa*.
56. A omits this line.
57. B *po*.
58. B *por*.

Rig pa ngo sprod 143

kun gzhi zhes pa'i ming du btags:[59] la las tha mal shes[60] pa'i[61] ming du btags: 'di nyid mngon sum[62] mdzub[63] btsugs[64] ngo sprod na: 'das pa'i rtog pa rjes med yal ba'i rting[65]: ma 'ongs rtog[66] pa ma shar[67] so ma la: da lta[68] bzo med rang lugs gnas pa'i dus: tha mal rang ga'i[69] dus kyi shes pa la[70]: rang gyis rang la[71] gcer gyis[72] bltas pa'i tshe: bltas pas mthong rgyu med pa'i gsal le ba: rig pa mngon sum[73] rjen pa hrig ge ba: cir yang grub med stong pa sang nge ba[74]: gsal stong gnyis su med pa'i yer re ba: rtag pa ma yin cir yang grub pa med: chad pa ma yin gsal[75] le hrig ge ba: gcig tu ma yin du mar rig cing gsal: du mar ma grub dbyer med ro gcig dang: gzhan na[76] med de[77] rang rig 'di nyid do[78]:

---

59. B inverts the last two lines.
60. A *zhes*.
61. B *pa*.
62. A *don gsum*. B *dngos su*. RN *mngon sum*.
63. A *'jug*. B *'dzub*.
64. A *tshul*.
65. A *gsal por stong* instead of *yal ba'i rting*.
66. A *rtogs*.
67. A *skyes*.
68. B *de ltar*.
69. A *gis*. B *gi*. RN *ga'i*.
70. B *ni*.
71. B *rang la rang gyis*.
72. A *gyi*.
73. B inserts *du*.
74. A *grub pa med pa'i stong sang nge* instead of *grub med stong pa sang nge ba*.
75. B *gsal*.
76. A *nas*.
77. A *pa*.
78. A *ni*.

dngos po'i gnas lugs don gyi ngo sprad de[79]: 'di la sku gsum dbyer med gcig tu[80] tshang: cir yang ma grub stong pa chos kyi sku: stong pa'i rang mdangs gsal ba longs sku yin: 'gag med cir yang 'char ba sprul pa'i sku: gsum ka gcig tu tshang ba ngo bo nyid: 'di nyid mdzub btsugs[81] btsan thabs ngo sprod[82] na: da lta rang gi shes pa 'di ka yin: ma bcos rang gsal 'di ka yin pa la: sems nyid ma rtogs bya ba ci la zer: 'di la bsgom[83] rgyu ci yang med pa la: bsgoms pas[84] ma byung bya ba ci la zer: rig pa mngon sum 'di ka yin pa la: rang sems ma rnyed bya ba ci la zer: gsal rig rgyun chad med pa 'di ka la: sems ngo ma mthong bya ba ci la zer: yid kyi bsam mkhan kho rang yin pa la: btsal bas[85] ma rnyed bya ba ci la zer: 'di la bya rgyu ci yang med pa la: byas pas ma byung bya ba ci la zer: ma bcos rang sar bzhag pas chog pa la: gnas su ma btub bya ba ci la zer: byar med cog ge bzhag[86] pas chog pa la: de la ma nus bya ba ci la zer: gsal rig stong gsum dbyer med lhun grub la: bsgrubs[87] pas ma grub[88] bya ba ci la zer: rgyu rkyen med par rang byung lhun grub la: rtsol bas ma nus bya ba ci la zer: rtog[89] pa shar grol dus mnyam yin pa la: gnyen pos ma thub bya ba ci la zer: da[90] lta'i shes pa 'di ka yin pa la: 'di la mi shes bya ba ci la zer: sems nyid stong pa gzhi med yin par nges: rang sems dngos

---

79. A sprod 'di. B sprod do. RN sprad de.
80. A la.
81. A 'jug tshul. B 'dzub tshugs.
82. A sprad.
83. A, B sgom.
84. B sgom pa.
85. A yang.
86. A, B zhag.
87. B sgrub.
88. A, B grub.
89. B rtogs.
90. A de.

med nam mkha' stong pa[91] 'dra: 'dra'am mi 'dra rang gi[92] sems la ltos: stong pa phyal chad[93] lta ba[94] ma yin par: rang byung ye shes ye nas gsal bar nges: rang byung rang gsal[95] nyi ma'i snying po 'dra: 'dra'am mi 'dra rang gi[96] sems la ltos: rig pa ye nas[97] rgyun chad med par nges:[98] rgyun chad med par chu yi[99] gzhung dang 'dra: 'dra'am mi 'dra rang gi sems la ltos[100]: rnam rtog[101] 'gyu[102] dran ngos bzung[103] med par nges: 'gyu[104] ba dngos med bar snang ser bu 'dra: 'dra'am mi 'dra rang gi sems la ltos[105]: cir snang thams cad rang snang yin par nges: snang ba[106] rang snang me long gzugs brnyan[107] 'dra: 'dra'am mi 'dra rang gi sems la ltos[108]: mtshan ma thams cad rang sar grol bar nges: rang byung rang grol bar snang sprin dang 'dra: 'dra'am mi 'dra rang gi sems la ltos[109]: sems las ma gtogs gzhan na chos med pas:

91. B *stong pa dngos med nam mkha'* instead of *dngos med nam mkha' stong pa.*
92. B *gis.*
93. A *chad chod.* B *chal chad.* RN *phyal chad.*
94. B *chad lta* instead of *lta ba.*
95. A *la.*
96. A *gis.*
97. A, B *shes.* RN *nas.*
98. B inserts *rig pa.*
99. A *chu'i.*
100. B *bltos.*
101. A *sna tshogs.*
102. A *rgyu.* B *'gyur.*
103. A *zungs.*
104. B *'gyur.*
105. B *bltos.*
106. A *bar.*
107. B *brnyen.*
108. B *bltos.*
109. B *bltos.*

lta ba blta[110] rgyu gzhan na chos med do:[111] sems las ma gtogs gzhan na chos med pas[112]: sgom pa bsgom rgyu gzhan na chos med do:[113] sems las ma gtogs[114] gzhan na chos med pas[115]: spyod pa spyad[116] rgyu gzhan na chos med do: sems las[117] ma gtogs[118] gzhan na chos med pas[119]: dam tshig bsrung rgyu gzhan na chos med do: sems las ma gtogs[120] gzhan na chos med pas[121]: 'bras bu bsgrub[122] rgyu gzhan na chos med do: yang ltos yang ltos rang gi sems la ltos: phyi rol nam mkha'i dbyings la[123] phar bltas pas: sems ni[124] 'phro ba'i 'phro sa mi 'dug na: nang du rang gi sems la tshur bltas pas: rtog pas[125] 'phro ba'i 'phro mkhan mi 'dug[126] na: rang sems phra phro[127] med pa'i gsal[128] le ba: rang rig[129] 'od gsal stong pa chos kyi sku: sprin med dvangs pa mkha' la[130] nyi shar 'dra:

---

110. B *lta*.
111. A omits these two lines.
112. A *do*.
113. A *sems las bhai ba bhai rgyu ga na yod:*.
114. A, B *rtogs*.
115. A *do*.
116. A, B *spyod*.
117. A *la*.
118. A, B *rtogs*.
119. A *do*.
120. A *rtogs*.
121. A *do*.
122. A, B *sgrub*.
123. A *su*.
124. B *'di*.
125. B *pa*.
126. B *gda'*.
127. B *'phra 'phro*.
128. B *sal*.
129. B *sems*.
130. A *nam mkha'i* instead of *mkha' la*.

Rig pa ngo sprod

rnam rtog[131] mi mnga' cir yang sa ler[132] mkhyen: 'di don rtogs dang ma rtogs khyad par che: gdod nas ma skyes rang byung 'od gsal 'di: pha ma med pa'i rig pa'i khye'u chung mtshar[133]: sus kyang ma byas rang byung ye shes mtshar[134]: skye ma myong zhing 'chi rgyu med pas[135] mtshar: mngon sum gsal yang[136] mthong mkhan med pas[137] mtshar: 'khor bar 'khyams kyang[138] ngan du mi 'gro[139] mtshar: sangs rgyas thob kyang[140] bzang du mi 'gro mtshar: kun la yod kyang ngo ma[141] shes pas mtshar: 'di bzhag[142] 'bras bu gzhan zhig[143] re bas[144] mtshar: rang nyid yin yang[145] gzhan du[146] btsal bas[147] mtshar: e ma: da lta'i rig pa dngos med gsal ba 'di: 'di ka lta ba kun gyi yang rtse yin: dmigs med khyab gdal[148] blo[149] dang bral ba 'di: 'di ka sgom pa kun gyi[150] yang

---

131. A *par*.
132. B *sal le*.
133. B *'tshar*.
134. B *'tshar*.
135. A *pa*.
136. A *kyang*.
137. A *pa'i*.
138. B *yang*.
139. B *ma song*.
140. A *mthong yang*.
141. A *mi*.
142. A *gzhan*.
143. A *cig*.
144. A *ba*.
145. A *kyang*.
146. B *zhig*.
147. A *rtsal ba*.
148. A *brdal*.
149. A *kun*.
150. B *gyis*.

rtse yin: ma bcos 'dzin med[151] lhug par 'jog[152] pa 'di: 'di ka spyod pa kun gyi yang rtse yin:[153] ma btsal[154] ye nas lhun gyis grub pa 'di: 'di ka 'bras bu kun gyi[155] yang rtse yin: nor ba med pa'i thig[156] chen bzhi bstan pa[157]: lta ba nor ba med pa'i thig[158] chen ni[159]: da lta'i shes pa gsal[160] le 'di yin pas: gsal la[161] mi nor bas na thig ces[162] bya: sgom pa[163] nor ba med pa'i thig[164] chen ni[165]: da lta'i shes pa gsal[166] le[167] 'di yin pas: gsal la mi nor bas na thig ces[168] bya: spyod pa nor ba med pa'i thig[169] chen ni: da lta'i shes pa[170] gsal le[171] 'di yin pas: gsal la[172] mi nor bas na thig[173] ces[174] bya: 'bras bu nor ba

---

151. A *'jig rten*. RN *'dzin med*.
152. A *brjod*. RN *'jog*.
153. B omits these two lines.
154. B *bcos*.
155. B *gyis*.
156. A, B *theg*. RN *thig*.
157. B *stan pas*.
158. A, B *theg*. RN *thig*.
159. A *'di*.
160. B *sal*.
161. B *ba*.
162. A, B *theg zhes*. RN *thig*.
163. A *bhai ba* instead of *sgom pa*.
164. A, B *theg*.
165. A *'di*.
166. B *sa*.
167. A *can*.
168. A, B *theg zhes*.
169. A, B *theg*.
170. A *ye shes*.
171. A *can*.
172. B *ba*.
173. A, B *theg*.
174. B *zhes*.

med pa'i thig[175] chen[176] ni: da lta'i shes pa gsal[177] le 'di yin
pas: gsal la mi nor bas na thig[178] ces bya: mi 'gyur ba yi gzer
chen bzhi[179] bstan[180] pa: lta ba 'gyur ba med pa'i gzer chen
ni[181]: da lta'i shes rig gsal le 'di ka yin: dus gsum brtan[182]
pa'i phyir na gzer zhes bya[183]: sgom pa 'gyur ba med pa'i
gzer chen ni: da lta'i shes rig gsal le 'di ka yin: dus gsum
brtan[184] pa'i phyir na gzer zhes bya[185]: spyod pa 'gyur ba
med pa'i gzer chen ni: da lta'i shes rig gsal[186] le 'di ka yin:
dus gsum brtan[187] pa'i phyir na gzer zhes bya[188]: 'bras bu
'gyur ba med pa'i gzer chen ni: da lta'i shes rig gsal le 'di
ka yin: dus gsum brtan[189] pa'i phyir na gzer zhes bya[190]:
dus gsum gcig tu gnas[191] pa'i man ngag ni[192]: sngar rjes mi
bcad[193] 'das pa'i 'dus shes dor[194]: phyis mdun[195] mi bsu yid

---

175. A, B *theg*.
176. A *can*.
177. B *sal*.
178. A, B *theg*.
179. A *gzhi*.
180. A, B *brtan*.
181. A *'di*.
182. A *bstan*.
183. A *bya'o*.
184. A *bstan*. B *brten*.
185. A *bya'o*.
186. B *sal*.
187. A *bstan*. B *brten*.
188. A *bya'o*.
189. A *bstan*.
190. A *bya'o*.
191. A *bstan*.
192. B *'di*.
193. A *spyad*.
194. A *bor*.
195. B *phyi bsdun*.

kyi[196] 'brel thag bcad: da lta 'dzin med nam mkha'i ngang la gzhag: bsgom[197] du med de ci yang mi sgom zhing: yengs su med de[198] yengs med dran pa bsten[199]: sgom[200] med yengs med ngang la gcer gyis ltos[201]: rang rig rang shes[202] rang gsal lhang nge ba: shar ba de ka byang chub sems zhes bya'o[203]: bsgom[204] du med de shes bya'i yul las 'das: yengs su med de ngo bo nyid kyis[205] gsal: snang stong rang grol gsal stong chos kyi sku: sangs rgyas lam gyis ma[206] bsgrubs[207] mngon gyur pas[208]: rdo rje sems dpa' dus 'dir[209] mthong ba yin: mthar thug[210] zad sar skyel ba'i gdams pa ni: lta ba mi mthun rgya che grangs mang yang: rang rig sems nyid[211] rang byung ye shes la: 'di la blta[212] bya lta[213] byed gnyis su med: lta ba ma ltos[214] lta ba'i[215] mkhan po tshol: lta mkhan

---

196. A kyis.
197. A, B sgom.
198. B pa'i.
199. A pas bstan.
200. A bhai.
201. B bltos.
202. B shes pa instead of rang shes.
203. B shes bya.
204. A bhai. B sgom.
205. A, B kyi.
206. A, B mi.
207. A sgrub.
208. B pa.
209. A 'di.
210. A mtha' drug.
211. A 'di.
212. A lta.
213. B blta.
214. A lta'am lta na. B lta ba ma lta.
215. B mkhan.

kho rang btsal bas ma rnyed na[216]: de'i[217] tshe lta ba zad sar 'khyol[218] ba yin: lta ba'i phugs kyang de ka[219] rang la thug: lta ba blta[220] rgyu ci yang med pa la: ye med stong pa phyal bar[221] ma song bar[222]: da lta rang gi[223] shes pa gsal le ba: rtogs[224] pa chen po'i lta ba de ka yin: rtogs dang ma rtogs de la gnyis su med: sgom[225] pa mi mthun rgya che grangs mang yang: rang rig tha mal shes[226] pa[227] zang thal la: bsgom[228] bya dang ni sgom byed gnyis su med:[229] sgom pa ma sgoms[230] sgom pa'i[231] mkhan po tshol:[232] sgom pa'i[233] mkhan po btsal bas ma rnyed na: de'i[234] tshe sgom pa zad sar 'khyol ba yin: sgom pa'i[235] phugs kyang de ka rang la thug[236]: sgom pa bya[237] rgyu ci yang med pa la: byin rmugs

---

216. A *pas*. B *pa*.
217. B *de*.
218. A *skyel*.
219. A *ga*.
220. A, B *lta*.
221. B *par*.
222. A *bas*. B *ba*.
223. A *rig*.
224. A *rdzogs*.
225. A *bsgom*.
226. B *shel*.
227. A *shes pa tha mal*.
228. B *sgom*.
229. A *bhai bya bhai byed gnyis su med pa la:*.
230. B *bsgom*.
231. B *mkhan*.
232. A *bhai dang mi bhai ba'i mkhan po tshol:*.
233. A *bha ba'i*.
234. B *de*.
235. A *bhai ba'i*.
236. A *thugs*.
237. A *bhai bya bhai* instead of *sgom pa bya*.

thibs[238] rgod dbang du ma song bar: da lta ma bcos shes pa gsal le ba: ma bcos mnyam par bzhag[239] pa'i[240] bsam gtan yin: gnas dang mi gnas de la gnyis su med: spyod pa mi mthun rgya che grangs mang yang: rang rig ye shes thig le nyag gcig la[241]: spyad[242] bya dang ni spyod byed gnyis su med: spyod pa ma spyod spyod mkhan de nyid[243] tshol: spyod mkhan de nyid btsal bas ma rnyed na: de'i[244] tshe spyod pa zad sar 'khyol ba yin: spyod pa'i phugs kyang de ka rang la thug: spyod pa bya rgyu ci yang[245] med pa la: bag chags[246] 'khrul pa'i dbang du ma song bar: da lta'i shes pa ma bcos rang gsal la: bcos bslad[247] blang dor gang yang mi byed pa[248]: de ka rnam par dag pa'i spyod pa yin: dag dang ma dag de la gnyis su med: 'bras bu mi mthun rgya che grangs mang yang: rang rig sems nyid sku gsum lhun grub la: bsgrub bya dang ni sgrub[249] byed gnyis su med: 'bras bu ma sgrubs sgrub[250] mkhan de nyid[251] tshol: sgrub[252] mkhan de nyid btsal bas ma rnyed na: de'i[253] tshe 'bras bu zad sar

---

238. A *gti mug 'thib* instead of *byin rmugs thibs*.
239. B *gzhag*.
240. A *pa*.
241. B *yin*.
242. B *spyod*.
243. A *nged kyi* instead of *de nyid*.
244. B *de*.
245. A *ye nas* instead of *ci yang*.
246. B *dgag sgrub* instead of *bag chags*.
247. A *slad*.
248. A *par*.
249. B *bsgrub*.
250. B *bsgrubs*.
251. A *'bras bu sgrub mkhan de nyid nged kyi* instead of *'bras bu ma sgrubs sgrub mkhan de nyid*.
252. A, B *bsgrub*.
253. B *de*.

'khyol ba yin: 'bras bu'i phugs kyang de ka rang la thug: 'bras bu bsgrub rgyu ci yang[254] med pa la: spang blang[255] re dogs dbang du ma song bar: da lta'i shes rig rang gsal lhun grub la: mngon gyur[256] sku gsum rang la[257] rtogs pa nyid: ye sangs rgyas pa'i 'bras bu de[258] nyid do: rtag[259] chad mtha' brgyad bral ba'i rig pa 'di: gang gi mthar ma lhung bas[260] dbu ma zer: dran rig rgyun chad med pas[261] rig pa zer: stong pa rig pa'i snying po can yin pas: de phyir bde gshegs snying po'i[262] ming du btags: 'di don shes na shes bya kun gyi rab[263]: de phyir shes rab pha rol phyin yang zer: blo 'das mtha' dang ye nas bral ba yi[264]: de phyir phyag rgya chen po'i[265] ming du btags: de nyid[266] rtogs dang ma rtogs khyad par las: 'khor 'das bde sdug kun gyi gzhir[267] gyur pas: de phyir kun gzhi zhes pa'i ming du btags: bzo[268] med tha[269] mal rang gar[270] gnas dus kyi[271]: shes pa gsal le hrig ge 'di ka[272] la: tha

254. A 'bras bu ci yod sgrub rgyu instead of 'bras bu sgrub rgyu ci yang.
255. A blangs.
256. A 'gyur.
257. B gsal.
258. A nyid.
259. A rtags.
260. A ba'i.
261. A par.
262. B po.
263. A kun gyis rab tu phyin instead of shes bya kun gyi rab.
264. A ba'i phyir instead of ba yi.
265. B por.
266. A, B phyir. RN nyid.
267. A gzhi.
268. A bzang.
269. B mtha'.
270. A mkhar. B khar.
271. A kyis.
272. A nyid.

mal shes pa zhes pa'i[273] ming du btags: bzang rtog snyan ming mang po ci btags kyang: don la da lta'i shes rig 'di ka las: 'di min[274] gzhan las[275] lhag pa su 'dod pa: glang po rnyed[276] kyang rjes 'tshol[277] de bzhin du[278]: stong gsum thog tu[279] 'brang[280] yang[281] rnyed mi srid: sems las ma gtogs[282] sangs rgyas rnyed mi srid: 'di ngo ma shes phyi rol sems btsal yang: rang gis[283] gzhan 'tshol rang nyid ci[284] phyir rnyed: dper na glen pa gcig[285] gis[286] mi mang khrod: lad mo[287] byas pas[288] rang nyid dor[289] nas su: rang ngo ma shes gzhan[290] du 'tshol[291] ba yang: rang gis[292] gzhan du[293] 'khrul pa de bzhin no: dngos po gshis kyi gnas lugs ma mthong bas: snang ba sems su ma shes 'khor bar gol[294]: rang sems sangs rgyas ma

273. B *'di ka* instead of *zhes pa'i*.
274. A *man*. B *ming*.
275. B *nas*.
276. B *rnyad*.
277. B *tshol*.
278. A *ji bzhin no*.
279. B *thags su*.
280. A *dran*. B *bran*. RN *'brang*.
281. A *kyang*.
282. A *rtog*.
283. B *gi*.
284. B *ci'i*.
285. A *cig*.
286. B *gi*.
287. A *ltas mos*. B *bltas mo*. RN *lad mo*.
288. B *bstas byas* instead of *byas pas*.
289. B *stor*.
290. A *bzhin*.
291. B *tshol*.
292. B *gi*.
293. B *'tshol*.
294. A *grol*.

Rig pa ngo sprod

rtogs[295] myang 'das bsgribs[296]: 'khor 'das gnyis la rig dang ma rig gi[297]: skad cig gcig gi[298] bar las[299] bye brag med: rang gi[300] sems las[301] gzhan du mthong bas 'khrul: 'khrul dang ma 'khrul ngo bo gcig pa ste: 'gro la sems rgyud gnyis su ma grub pas: sems nyid ma bcos rang sar bzhag[302] pas grol: 'khrul pa de nyid sems su ma rig na[303]: chos nyid don de nam yang ma[304] rtogs pas: rang byung rang shar[305] rang gis rang la[306] blta: snang ba 'di dag dang po gang nas[307] byung: bar du gar gnas mtha' mar[308] gang du 'gro:[309] bltas pas dper na rdzings kyi[310] bya rog bzhin[311]: rdzings[312] nas 'phur yang[313] rdzings[314] las logs na[315] med: de bzhin snang ba sems las

---

295. A *mthong*.
296. A *sgribs*.
297. A, B *gis*.
298. A, B *gis*.
299. A *la*.
300. A, B *gis*.
301. A *la*.
302. B *gzhag*.
303. A *ni*.
304. A, B *mi*.
305. A *rang shar rang byung* instead of *rang byung rang shar*.
306. B *rang la rang gis* instead of *rang gis rang la*.
307. A *las*.
308. B *tha ma*.
309. A *bar du gang las gnas shing mtha' mar gar 'gro ba:*.
310. A, B *rdzing gi*. RN *rdzings kyi*.
311. B *gis*.
312. A, B *rdzing*.
313. A *phur kyang*.
314. A, B *rdzing*.
315. A, B *log pa*. RN *logs na*.

shar ba'i phyir[316]: rang gi[317] sems las shar zhing sems su[318] grol: sems nyid kun shes kun rig stong gsal 'di: gdod nas gsal stong dbyer med nam mkha' ltar: rang byung ye shes mngon sum gsal ba ru: gtan la phebs pa de ka chos nyid do: yin pa'i rtags[319] ni snang srid thams cad kun[320]: rang gi sems su rig cing sems nyid 'di[321]: rig cing gsal bas[322] nam mkha' lta bur rtogs: chos nyid mtshon pa'i nam mkha' dper bzhag kyang[323]: re zhig phyogs tsam mtshon pa'i brda' tsam ste: sems nyid rig bcas stong[324] pa cir yang gsal: nam mkha' rig med stong pa bem stong ste[325]: de phyir sems don nam mkha' mtshon du med: yengs su med kyis[326] de ka'i ngang la zhog[327]: snang ba kun rdzob sna tshogs 'di dag[328] kyang: gcig kyang bden par ma grub 'jig pa bzhin: dper na snang srid 'khor 'das thams cad kun: rang gi[329] sems nyid gcig pu'i[330] mthong snang yin: gang tshe rang gi sems rgyud 'gyur tsam na: phyi ru[331] 'gyur ba de yi[332] mthong snang 'byung:

---

316. A *ba bzhin*.
317. A *gis*.
318. B *las*.
319. B *pa dag*.
320. A *kyang*.
321. A *ni*.
322. B *ba*.
323. B *nas*.
324. A *stongs*.
325. A *stongs te*.
326. B *kyi*.
327. A, B *bzhog*.
328. B *'di dag sna tshogs*.
329. B *rig*.
330. B *gi*.
331. B *rgyu*.
332. A *de'i*.

Rig pa ngo sprod

des na thams cad sems kyi mthong snang ste[333]: 'gro ba rigs drug so so'i[334] snang bar mthong: phyi rol[335] mu stegs rtag chad gnyis su mthong: theg pa rim dgu[336] so so'i lta bar mthong: sna tshogs mthong zhing sna tshogs mi gcig pa[337]: tha dad gzung bas so sor[338] zhen[339] pas 'khrul: snang ba thams cad sems su rig pas na[340]: mthong snang shar yang 'dzin med sangs rgyas yin: snang ba ma 'khrul 'dzin pas 'khrul ba yin: 'dzin rtog sems su shes na rang[341] gis grol: cir snang thams cad sems kyi snang ba yin: snod kyi 'jig rten bem[342] por snang ba'ang[343] sems: bcud kyi sems can rigs drug snang ba'ang[344] sems: mtho ris[345] lha mi'i[346] bde bar[347] snang ba'ang[348] sems: ngan song gsum gyi sdug bsngal snang ba'ang sems: ma rig nyon mongs dug lngar[349] snang ba'ang sems: rang byung ye shes rig par[350] snang ba'ang sems: ngan rtog[351]

---

333. B *yin*.
334. A *sor*.
335. A *ru*.
336. B *theg rim dgu'i*.
337. A *gsal ba bzhin* instead of *mi gcig pa*.
338. A *so'i*.
339. B *gzhen*.
340. A *pa ni*.
341. B *ngang*.
342. B *ben*.
343. B *ba*.
344. B *ba*.
345. A *rigs*.
346. A *ma'i*.
347. A *ba*. B *ba'ang*.
348. B *ba*.
349. A *lnga*.
350. A *pa*.
351. B *rtogs*.

'khor ba'i bag chags snang ba'ang sems:³⁵² bzang rtog myang 'das zhing khams³⁵³ snang ba'ang sems: bdud dang 'dre yi³⁵⁴ bar chad snang ba'ang sems: lha dang dngos grub legs par snang ba'ang sems: rnam par rtog³⁵⁵ pa sna tshogs snang ba'ang sems: mi rtog rtse gcig gnas³⁵⁶ par snang ba'ang sems: dngos po mtshan ma'i kha dog snang ba'ang sems: mtshan med spros pa med par³⁵⁷ snang ba'ang³⁵⁸ sems: gcig dang du ma gnyis med snang ba'ang sems: yod med gang du ma grub snang ba'ang³⁵⁹ sems: sems las ma gtogs³⁶⁰ snang ba gang yang med: sems nyid ma 'gags snang ba gang yang 'char: shar yang rgya mtsho'i³⁶¹ chu dang chu rlabs bzhin: gnyis su med de sems kyi³⁶² ngang du grol: gtags³⁶³ bya ma 'gags ming 'dogs ci btags kyang: don la sems nyid³⁶⁴ gcig las yod ma yin: gcig po de yang gzhi med rtsa bral yin: gang gi phyogs su³⁶⁵ mthong ba gcig kyang med: dngos por³⁶⁶ ma mthong cir yang³⁶⁷ grub pa med: stong par ma mthong rig cing gsal ba'i mdangs³⁶⁸: so sor ma mthong gsal

---

352. A omits this line.
353. A *mya ngan 'das shing* instead of *myang 'das zhing khams*.
354. A *'dre'i*.
355. A *dag*.
356. B *sgom*.
357. A *pa*.
358. B *mtshan ma med cing spros pa med pa'ang* instead of *mtshan med spros pa med par snang ba'ang*.
359. B *pa yang*.
360. A *rtogs*.
361. B *mtsho yi*.
362. B *nyid*.
363. A, B *btags*.
364. A *ni*.
365. B *su'ang*.
366. A, B *po*.
367. B *gcig kyang*.
368. A *mdang*.

Rig pa ngo sprod 159

stong[369] dbyer med ngang[370]: da lta rang gi shes pa gsal hrig ge[371]: yin[372] par byas kyang de nyid byed mi shes: rang bzhin med kyang mngon sum nyams[373] su myong: 'di nyid nyams su blangs na kun grol te[374]: dbang po dag la rno[375] rtul[376] med par rtogs: til dang 'o ma mar gyi rgyu yin kyang: ma bsrubs[377] ma btsir[378] khu ba[379] mi 'byung ltar: 'gro kun sangs rgyas snying po dngos yin kyang: nyams su ma blangs sems can sangs mi rgya: nyams su blangs na ba lang[380] rdzi yang grol: bshad mi shes kyang mngon sum gtan la phebs: rang gis[381] kha ru myong ba'i bu ram la: gzhan gyis[382] de yi[383] ro bshad mi dgos bzhin[384]: 'di nyid ma rtogs paṇḍi ta yang 'khrul: theg dgu'i bshad pa shes bya mkhas gyur kyang: ma mthong rgyang gi[385] gtam rgyud[386] bsnyad[387] pa bzhin: sangs rgyas la ni skad cig nyer ma reg[388]: 'di nyid rtogs na

---

369. B *stong gsal*.
370. A *dang*.
371. B *rig de*.
372. B *min*.
373. A *nyams su dngos* instead of *mngon sum nyams*.
374. B *kyang grol* instead of *grol te*.
375. A *blo*.
376. A, B *brtul*.
377. A *bslug*. B *srubs*.
378. B *rtsir*.
379. B *mar khu*.
380. B *glangs*.
381. B *gi*.
382. B *gyi*.
383. A, B *de'i*.
384. A *shing*.
385. B *gzhan gyi*.
386. B *rgyus*.
387. A *bsnyegs*. B *bshad*. RN *bsnyad*.
388. B *mthong*.

dge sdig rang sar grol: 'di nyid ma rtogs dge sdig gang spyad kyang: mtho ris[389] ngan song 'khor ba las mi 'phags[390]: rang sems stong gsal[391] ye shes rtogs tsa[392] na: dge sdig phan gnod[393] gang yang ma grub pas[394]: bar snang stong par chu mi[395] chags pa bzhin: stong pa nyid la dge sdig yul ma grub: des na rang rig mngon sum gcer mthong du[396]: gcer mthong rang grol 'di nyid rab tu zab: de phyir rang rig 'di la[397] 'dris par gyis[398]: zab rgya[399]: e ma:[400] rig pa ngo sprod gcer mthong rang grol 'di[401]: ma 'ongs phyi rabs snyigs ma'i skal ldan[402] don: rgyud lung man ngag rang gi nyams myong[403] kun: dgongs[404] pa mdor bsdus nyung gsal[405] 'di sbyar ro: da lta spel phangs[406] rin chen gter du sbos[407]: ma 'ongs las 'phro can dang 'phrad par shog: sa ma yā: rgya rgya rgya: rig pa

---

389. A *rigs*.
390. A *bsags*.
391. A *pa*.
392. A *tsam*.
393. A *yon*.
394. A *po*.
395. A, B *mig*. RN *mi*.
396. B *phog tu*.
397. A *nyid*.
398. A *bgyi*.
399. B *zab: rgya rgya rgya:*.
400. A, B omit :.
401. A *te*.
402. A *sems can*.
403. A *mos pa*.
404. A *dgos*.
405. A *ba*.
406. A *yang*.
407. A *sbas*.

Rig pa ngo sprod

mngon sum ngo sprod pa'i[408] bstan bcos:[409] gcer mthong rang grol zhes bya ba: u[410] rgyan gyi mkhan po padma 'byung gnas kyis[411] sbyar ba[412]: 'khor ba ma stong bar du ma[413] rdzogs so:[414]

---

408. B inserts:.
409. B omits:.
410. A *o*.
411. B *kyi*.
412. B inserts *rdzogs so*.
413. B omits this line.
414. B inserts :*sa ma yā: rgya rgya rgya: oṁ vajra satva hūṁ āḥ tadya thāḥ oṁ pañtsi grī ya ā vā bho dha ni ye svā hāḥ bkra shis//*

Appendix 4.

KUN BYED RGYAL PO

(1) /kye sems dpa' chen po rdo rje[1] khyod nyon cig /nga ni ye nas rang 'byung[2] ye shes te//nga ni ye nas chos kun snying po yin//nga ni kun byed rgyal po byang chub sems//nga yi mtshan 'di[3] sems dpas[4] rtogs par gyis//nga yi mtshan 'di[5] sems dpas rtogs gyur[6] na//chos rnams thams cad ma lus rtogs 'gyur gyis/ (Chap. 4)

(2) /nga zhes bya ba snying po ste//chos rnams kun gyi snying po yin//rang 'byung zhes ni bya ba ni//rgyu rkyen med pa'i snying po bas//rtsol sgrub[7] kun las 'das pa yin//ye shes zhes ni bya ba ni//'gag pa med cing ma bsgribs pas//chos kun ma lus ston par byed//nga ni byang chub sems la bya//

---

1. A omits *rdo rje*.
2. A, B *byung*.
3. B *ni*.
4. C *dpa'*.
5. B *ni*.
6. C *'gyur*.
7. A *bsgrub*.

Kun byed rgyal po

ye nas bya ba'i don 'di ni//thog ma nyid nas gnas pa'i don//
chos kun zhes ni bya ba ni//ston pa kun kyang chos nyid la/
/bstan pa kun kyang chos nyid yin//'khor gnas dus[8] kyang[9]
chos nyid de[10]//chos nyid ma yin gcig[11] kyang med//snying
po bya ba'i don 'di[12] ni//thams cad 'byung ba'i snying po
ste//byang chub sems kyi rang bzhin las[13]//ston pa gsum
yang de las byung//bstan pa gsum yang de las byung//'khor
gnas dus kyang de las byung//thams cad 'byung ba'i snying
por bshad//nga ni snying po sems nyid kyis//chos rnams ma
lus kun byed de[14]/ [. . .] /byed ces bya ba mkhan po ste//ston
pa dang ni bstan pa dang//'khor gnas dus ni kun byed pas//
rang 'byung ye shes mkhan po yin//rgyal po zhes ni bya ba
ni//snying po rang 'byung ye shes de//byed pa'i mkhan po
kun las rgyal//chos rnams byed mkhan kun las rgyal//byang
ba'i[15] don ni 'di lta ste//snying po byang chub sems de ni//
rang 'byung ye nas rnam dag pas//kun byed rgyal pos byas
pa kun//kun bzang nyid du rnam dag pas//byang zhes bya
bar bshad pa yin//chub ces bya ba 'di lta ste//snying po rang
'byung ye shes des//snang ba dang ni srid pa dang//snod
dang bcud kyis bsdus pa dang//dus gsum sangs rgyas thams
cad dang//khams gsum rgyud drug sems can dang//de bzhin
nyid ni thams cad la//kun la chub ste khyab par gnas//des
na chub ces bya bar bshad//sems kyi don ni 'di lta ste//
snying po rang 'byung ye shes des//snang srid snod bcud
thams cad la//'jug cing dbang sgyur[16] gsal bar gcod/ des na
sems zhes bya bar bshad//rgyu rkyen med pa'i snying po

---

8. A *kun*. B *dus kun*.
9. B *'ang*.
10. A, B *yin*.
11. C *cig*.
12. A, B *chos nyid*.
13. A, B *la*.
14. A *te*.
15. C *byed pa'i*.
16. A *bsgyur*.

des//kun la dbang sgyur[17] thams cad byed//kye sems dpa' chen po//nga yi rang bzhin rtogs gyur na//ston pa kun kyang rtogs 'gyur la[18]//bstan pa kun kyang rtogs par 'gyur rig / chos//'khor gyi bsam pa rig gyur[19] la//dus gnas kun kyang gcig 'gyur rig /chos rnams thams cad nga yin pas//nga yi rang bzhin 'di rig na//chos rnams thams cad rig gyur bas[20]// bya byed rtsol sgrub kun las 'das//mi rtsol lhun gyis grub par 'gyur zhes gsungs so/(Chap. 4)

(3)/nga yi rang bzhin ma bcos chos skur[21] grub//nga yi ngo bo ma bcos longs spyod rdzogs//nga yi thugs rje mngon phyung sprul sku gsum/(Chap. 19)

(4)/nga ni ston pa'i sgron ma byang chub sems//dus gsum sangs rgyas kun gyi snying po yin//khams gsum sems can kun gyi pha dang ma//snang srid snod bcud kun gyi rgyu yang yin//nga las ma byung ba[22] ni gcig[23] kyang med//nga ni mi gnas kun du khyab pa'i phyir//nga ni ye nas dus gsum sangs rgyas yin//nga ni mi rtog mnyam par gnas pa'i phyir/ /rtog med mnyam nyid chos sku ye sangs rgyas//nga yi ngo bo kun du longs spyod phyir//nga nyid longs spyod rdzogs skur ye sangs rgyas//nga nyid rang 'byung ye shes snang ba'i phyir/ /nga nyid thugs rje sprul skur mngon sangs rgyas/ (Chap. 41)

(5) /snang srid gnod bcud de[24] ltar snang ba las//nga la sku[25] yi ngo bo gzhan med pas//rang gi ngo bos 'chad cing ston pa

---

17. A *bsgyur*.
18. A *ba*.
19. A, B *'gyur*.
20. A, B *'gyur bas*. C *'gyur pas*.
21. A *sku*. C *kur*.
22. A *pa*.
23. C *cig*.
24. A, B *'di*.
25. C *ku*.

Kun byed rgyal po 165

yin/[. . .] /sa chu me rlung nam mkha'i sgra grag[26] dang//
rgyud drug sems can rnams kyi sgra tshig 'di//kun byed nga
yi gsung las gzhan med pas//tshig sgra don gyi bsdebs[27] bshad
de la bya/[. . .] /khams gsum rgyud drug sems can thams cad
dang//'byung chen lnga yi mi rtog mnyam nyid dang//chos
nyid mi skye mi rtog mi 'gag ste//kun byed nga yi thugs su
de las med/ (Chap. 36)

(6)/kye nga ni ston pa kun byed rgyal po la//ston pa rang
'byung rig pa'i ye shes las[28]//ma bsdus ston pa gsum yang
de la 'dus/ [. . .] /bstan pa brjod[29] bral rig pa mtshon[30] 'das la/
/bstan pa gsum yang de la 'dus te gnas[31]//ma bcos rig pa'i
gzhal yas 'og min na//gzhal yas gsum yang de la 'dus par
bshad//ji ltar snang ba'i chos rnams[32] thams cad kun//snying
po byang chub sems la[33] kun 'dus pas//'khor gsum dus gsum
kun du[34] 'dus par bshad//ma bsdus[35] rang bzhin 'du ba'i ye
shes ni//sdud[36] pa de las gzhan pa yod ma yin/ (Chap. 70)

(7)/rang rig ma nor blo yi tsad ma yis//ma bcos snying po'i
don la 'jug par byed/ (Chap. 72)

(8)/sangs rgyas sku dang ye shes yon tan dang//sems can lus
dang bag chags la sogs pa//snang srid snod[37] bcud bsdus pa
thams cad kun//byang chub sems kyi ngo bo ye nas yin//

---

26. B *grags*.
27. C *sdebs*.
28. A *la*.
29. C *rjod*.
30. B *mtshan*.
31. A *bstan*.
32. C *rnam*.
33. A *su*.
34. A *kun tu yang* instead of *gsum kun du*. B *kyang kun tu*.
35. B *'dus*. C *sdus*.
36. B *bsdus*.
37. C *gnod*.

sems las ma gtogs[38] pa yi chos rnams ni//nga las byung ba'i sangs rgyas sngar 'das la//kun byed rgyal po nga yis lung ma bstan//da ltar bzhugs dang slad kyis 'byon[39] pa la//kun byed rgyal po byang chub lung mi ston/ (Chap. 6)

(9)/nga nyid kun gyi mdun du mngon phyung[40] yang//sku gsum 'khor gyis rnam rtog grangs su rtogs/(Chap. 65)

(10)/chos kun rtsa ba byang chub sems su gcig /sangs rgyas sems can snang srid snod bcud kun//thams cad 'byung ba'i byang chub snying po la//gcig tu med las bgrangs na brjod mi lang/(Chap. 6)

(11)/rgyu ni lta ba sgom[41] pa byas pa yis//gang bsgoms[42] 'bras bu de thob 'dod pa ni//sgom[43] pa de yis 'bras bu thob pa med//thams cad ji bzhin pa yi chos yin pas//ji bzhin pa la 'chos par byed pa ni//brdzun[44] gyis bden pa bslus[45] pa[46] sdig re che/(Chap. 35)

(12)/rgyu dang 'bras bu yod zer smra byed pa//de ni rdzogs chen rtogs[47] pa'i don mi ldan//don dam kun rdzob gnyis su smra byed pa[48]//sgro dang skur pa[49] 'debs pa'i tshig yin te// de yis gnyis su med pa rtogs pa med//dus gsum sangs rgyas

---

38. C *rtogs*.
39. C *byon*.
40. C *byung*.
41. A *bsgom*.
42. C *sgoms*.
43. B *bsgom*.
44. C *rdzun*.
45. C *slus*.
46. B *pas*.
47. B *rtog*.
48. C *na*.
49. C *ba*.

rnams kyi rtogs[50] pa yang//gnyis su ma mthong rnal bzhag[51] gcig tu rtogs[52]/(Chap. 29)

(13)/kun byed rgyal po skye ba med par rtogs//chos kun rtsa ba kun byed nga nyid[53] de[54]//nga[55] nyid ma skyes dbyings su rtogs pas na//kun kyang skye med dbyings su rtogs par 'gyur/ (Chap. 58)

(14)/dus gsum gcig ste khyad par med//sngon med phyis med gdod nas 'byung/(Chap. 30)

(15)/kun byed byang chub nga yi rang bzhin las//ma btsal rang bzhin lhun gyis grub pa ni//rgyal ba kun gyi snying po sku gsum ste[56]//nga yi rang bzhin ma bcos chos skur[57] grub/ /nga yi ngo bo ma bcos longs spyod rdzogs//nga yi thugs rje mngon phyung sprul sku gsum//btsal nas grub pa'i 'bras bu bstan pa med/ (Chap. 19)

(16)/ye nas kun byed nyid kyis byas pa'i phyir//lam la mi bgrod sa la sbyong[58] mi byed//dam tshig mi srung[59] lta ba sgom[60] mi byed//byang chub chen po'i lam nas[61] kun 'byung[62] phyir//byang chub nyid la[63] byang chub nyid mi bgrod//

---

50. B *kyis rtog.*
51. A, B *gzhag.*
52. A *rtog.* C *nyid du 'dod* instead of *gcig tu rtogs.*
53. C *byang chub kun byed.*
54. A *do.*
55. C *de.*
56. C *to.*
57. A *sku.* C *kur.*
58. C *sbyongs.*
59. A *bsrung.* C *srun.*
60. A *bsgom.*
61. A, B *las.*
62. B *byung.*
63. B *las.*

bgrod sa byang chub nyid las med pa'i phyir//byang chub
nyid la byang chub nyid mi sbyong[64]//dam tshig rang bzhin
byang chub nyid yin pas//byang chub nyid la byang chub
nyid mi srung[65]//sgom[66] pa'i rang bzhin byang chub nyid yin
pas//byang chub nyid kyis nyid la bsgom[67] du med//lta ba'i
yul ni byang chub nyid yin pas//byang chub nyid kyis nyid
la[68] bltar[69] med phyir/(Chap. 8)

(17)/ji ltar snang ba'i chos rnams la//byang chub sems su ma
rtogs te//bcos zhing bsgrubs pas 'grub mi 'gyur//ma rtogs
bcos pas grub pa byed//bskal pa du ma'i grangs bgrangs
kyang//mi rtsol[70] bde ba[71] phrad mi 'gyur/[. . .]/de bzhin
'chos par byed pa yi//ston pas bden[72] tshul ji bstan yang//
nges lung ma yin drang lung yin/(Chap. 42)

(18)/kye nga las byung ba'i ston pa sku gsum gyis//mtshan
ma bsgom la[73] dga' ba'i gang zag la//rang rang gang ltar 'thad
pa'i lung bzhin du//bsgom du yod ces kun la lung du bstan/
(Chap. 70)

(19)/bskal[74] pa dpag tu med pa'i sngon rol nas//kun byed
byang chub nga la dad pa yi//las dang skal ldan shin tu rnal
'byor pa//lta ba bsgom[75] med dam tshig bsrung[76] du med//

---

64. C sbyongs.
65. A bsrung.
66. A, B bsgom.
67. C sgom.
68. A, B nyid la nyid kyis.
69. A ltar.
70. C brtsol.
71. A, B dang.
72. A sde.
73. B du.
74. C skal.
75. A, C sgom.
76. C gsung.

'phrin[77] las btsal[78] med lam la bgrod du med//sa la sbyang
med rgyu dang 'bras bu med//don dam dang ni kun rdzob
rnam gnyis med//bsgom[79] zhing bsgrub[80] tu med par mthong
ba dang//sems bskyed[81] med cing gnyen po med mthong ba[82]/
/kun byed sems kyi rang bzhin mthong ba yi//de lta bu yi
dgos ched bstan pa yin/ (Chap. 13)

(20)/kun byed nga yis theg gcig[83] bstan pa ni//btsal bas[84] grub
pa'i lung du ngas ma bstan[85]/(Chap. 19)

(21)/bya ba med pa'i don 'di ni//kun byed nga yi rang bzhin
te//nga la bya ba med pa ni//nga ni ye nas byas zin pas//
bya ba med pa'i chos nyid yin//chos nyid nga yi rang bzhin
las[86]//rang bzhin de la bya ru med//rang bzhin rang bzhin
bya ba de//bcos su med pa'i rang bzhin yin//bcos med byang
chub de la ni//sems dpa' rdo rje khyod ma 'chos//sems dpa'
rdo rjes[87] de 'chos na//kun byed nga la 'chos pa yin//ji ltar
snang ba'i chos rnams kun//kun byed nga yi rang bzhin yin/
/kye sems dpa' chen po khyod nyon cig /nga yi rang bzhin
'gyur med la//bsgoms na 'chos[88] shing bsgyur[89] ba yin//nga
ni ye nas lhun grub la//bsgrubs na nga la bcos pa yin//nga la
bgrod pas phyin pa med//nga la btsal bas[90] grub pa med//

77. C phrin.
78. A rtsal.
79. A sgom.
80. A, C sgrub.
81. C skyed.
82. A, B bas.
83. C cig.
84. C ba.
85. B bshad.
86. A, B pas.
87. A, B rje.
88. C mchos.
89. C rgyur.
90. C pas.

nga la sbyangs pas byang ba med//nga la ma lta yul med kyis// nga la ma bgrod lam med kyis//nga la ma sbyongs[91] sgrib med kyis//mi gnas dmigs pa'i yul dang bral//spros med bsam pa'i yul las 'das/(Chap. 44)

(22)/thams cad gcig[92] phyir nga la kun rdzogs te//rdzogs pa chen po nga la kun rdzogs pas//lta spyod 'phrin[93] las dam tshig sa lam ni//gong bshad bzhin du brtsal[94] zhing bsgrub[95] mi dgos//de ltar ma rig rtsol[96] sgrub byas gyur[97] na//rgyu 'bras 'das pa'i don dang 'gal gyur[98] nas//bya med bde chen de dang mi phrad[99] de//rtsol[100] sgrub nad kyis ma rig de zin 'gyur//de bas rgyu 'bras 'das pa'i rdzogs chen la//skal med rnams kyi spyod yul ma yin pas//rgyu dang 'bras bu'i chos la spyad par bya/ (Chap. 44)

(23)/kun byed nga yi rang bzhin gcig[101] pu la//'khor gyi 'dod pa rnams kyis[102] ming btags[103] pa//la las byang chub sems su ming btags la//la las chos kyi dbyings su ming yang btags// la las nam mkha'i khams su ming yang btags[104]//la las rang 'byung ye shes ming yang btags//la las chos kyi sku[105] ru ming yang btags//la las longs spyod rdzogs par ming yang btags/

---

91. A, B *sbyong*.
92. C *cig*.
93. C *phrin*.
94. A, B, C *btsal*.
95. A *sgrub*.
96. C *brtsol*.
97. C *'gyur*.
98. C *'gyur*.
99. A, B *'phrad*.
100. C *brtsol*.
101. C *cig*.
102. C *kyi*.
103. C *rtags*.
104. A *brtags*.
105. C *skur*.

Kun byed rgyal po

/la las sprul pa'i sku ru ming yang btags//la las sku gsung thugs su ming yang btags//la las thams cad mkhyen par ming yang btags//la las rnam pa thams cad ming yang btags//la las ye shes[106] bzhi dang gsum du btags//la las ye shes lnga ru ming btags la//la las dbyings dang ye shes ming btags pa// rang 'byung byang chub sems ni gcig la btags//rang 'byung nga la mthong tshad smras pa yin/(Chap. 50)

(24) /kye sems dpa' rdo rje ji bzhin nyid sgoms[107] shig /rtog[108] pa rang sar grol ba'i lta ba la//ma yengs rang bzhin bzhag[109] pas bya rtsol[110] med//kun kyang rang 'byung rang sar grol ba yin//kye sems dpa' rdo rje ji bzhin nyid sgoms[111] shig /rang lus ma[112] bcos[113] dbang po ma[114] btul[115] te//ngag kyang ma[116] bsdams[117] bya rtsol[118] byar yang med//sems kyang gar[119] btang[120] mi g.yo'i ngang la gzhag[121] (Chap. 73)

(25)/rdzogs chen lta ba bsgom[122] du med pa ni//kun byed nga yi sems kyi yon tan te//byang chub sems kyi che ba'i yon

---

106. A omits *ye shes*.
107. A *bsgoms*.
108. B, C *rtogs*.
109. A, B *gzhag*.
110. A *brtsal*. B, C *btsal*.
111. A *bsgoms*.
112. A, B, C *mi*.
113. A *bcom*.
114. A, B, C *mi*.
115. B *brtul*. C *rtul*.
116. A, B, C *mi*.
117. A, B, *bsdam*. C *gdams*.
118. A *brtsal*. B *btsal*.
119. C *gang*.
120. B *gtang*.
121. C *bzhag*.
122. A *sgom*.

tan gyis//brtsal[123] zhing bsgrub[124] pa'i bka' ba spyad[125] mi dgos//rgyu rkyen med pas btsal ba'i las mi dgos//'bras bu'i rang bzhin gzhan nas bsgrub[126] mi dgos//chos nyid rang yin sgom[127] pa bya mi dgos//ma skyes pas na 'jig pa'i gnyen[128] po med//gzhan la ma ltos sgom[129] gnas 'tshol[130] mi byed//nga la gang zhig sgom par byed pa des//bsgoms pa nyid kyis[131] nga dang phrad mi 'gyur//chos nyid mngon du phyung ba[132] nga yin pas//sdug bsngal mi skye rnam par spang mi dgos//rang 'byung[133] yin pas skye 'jig med pa'i phyir//ma rig rten 'brel dbang po dgag mi dgos/ (Chap. 45)

(26)/kye kun byed rgyal po byang chub sems nga[134] ni//chos rnams kun gyi lta ba'i me long ste//gsal la rang bzhin med par kun 'char bas/(Chap. 59)

(27)/nga med pa yi yul ni[135] gzhan med pas//lta ba bsgom du med par la yang bzlas//nga las gzhan du bsrung du med pa'i phyir//dam tshig bsrung du med par la yang bzlas//nga las gzhan du btsal du med pa'i phyir//'phrin[136] las btsal du[137] med par la yang bzlas[138]//nga las gzhan du gnas pa med pa'i phyir/

---

123. A, B, C btsal.
124. C sgrubs.
125. C cad.
126. A, C sgrub.
127. B bsgom.
128. A, B dngos.
129. B bsgom.
130. A, B, C tshol.
131. A kyi. B kyang.
132. A pa.
133. A, B byung.
134. C de.
135. A, B na.
136. C phrin.
137. A, B bya ru.
138. C 'das.

/sa la sbyang du med par la yang bzlas//nga la sgrib pa ye nas med pa'i phyir//rang 'byung ye shes yin par la yang bzlas[139]//nga ni ma skyes chos nyid yin pa'i phyir//phra ba chos nyid yin par la yang bzlas[140]//nga las gzhan du bgrod du med pa'i phyir//lam la bgrod du med par la yang bzlas//sangs rgyas sems can snang srid snod bcud kun//snying po byang chub nga las byung ba'i phyir//ye nas gnyis su med par la yang bzlas//rang 'byung ye shes gtan la 'bebs pa'i phyir// lung chen thog[141] 'bebs yin par la yang bzlas//chos rnams thams cad nga las med pa'i phyir//kun byed nga ni kun gyi la bzla'o[142]//nga ma shes pas[143] sgrib pa'i ngo bor bshad//nga las gzhan btsal gol sa byung ba yin/(Chap. 9)

(28)/kye kun byed rig pas dbang bsgyur[144] dgongs pa 'di// ngag gis smrar med dmigs pa'i yul las 'das//dran pa zhi zhing spros pa med pa ste//mkha' ltar khyab cing phyogs cha yongs kyis med/ (Chap. 75)

(29) /kun byed rgyal po byang chub sems nga ni//bstan pa kun gyi yang rtse yin par bshad//nga las byung ba'i ston pa sku gsum gyis//bstan[145] pa'i 'dul ba[146] mdo sde mngon pa dang//tan tra so so'i sde ni 'bum sde dang//bskyed[147] rdzogs gsang ba la sogs rtsol[148] sgrub can//kun kyang rtsol sgrub 'das pa nga la bgrod//rtsol sgrub nyid kyis 'das pa[149] nga mi

---

139. C 'das.
140. A bzla.
141. B thogs.
142. A zla'o.
143. A, B pa.
144. B sgyur. C rgyur.
145. C stan.
146. C pa.
147. C skyed.
148. C brtsol.
149. A pas.

mthong//des na bstan pa kun gyi yang rtse yin par bshad/ (Chap. 12)

(30)/kye sems dpa' chen po nyon cig /chos rnams thams cad thig le chen po'i rang bzhin yin[150] pas na//spros pa med cing bsdus[151] pa med//skye ba med cing 'gag pa med//'gog[152] pa med par de bzhin gnas//rnam par mi rtog snying po 'di// nam mkha' bzhin du ye gnas pas//rtog pa'i smra[153] bsam yul las 'das/ (Chap. 26)

(31)/des bas snang srid snod bcud thams cad kun//nam mkha'i ngang na mi gnas med pa bzhin//byang schub sems kyi klong chen yul che bas//sangs rgyas sems can snod bcud kun kyang gnas[154]/(Chap. 6)

(32)/de ltar bsgom[155] du med pa'i snying po la//ma yengs dran pas bzung[156] ba[157] man ngag yin/(Chap. 77)

(33)/ma bcos rnal ma kun gyi chos nyid yin//chos nyid las ni sangs rgyas gud na med//sangs rgyas ming du btags[158] pa bla dags yin//chos nyid bya ba gzhan med rang sems te// rang sems ma bcos chos kyi sku ru bshad//ma bcos pa la ye nas skye med pas//skye med don la brtsal[159] zhing bsgrub[160] tu med//brtsal[161] zhing bsgrubs[162] pas bya med 'grub mi 'gyur/ (Chap. 15)

---

150. A omits *yin*.
151. C *sdus*.
152. A *'gag*.
153. C *smras*.
154. A *snang srid snod bcud kun* instead of *snod bcud kun kyang gnas*.
155. C *sgom*.
156. B *gzung*.
157. A *bas*.
158. C *rtags*.
159. A, B *btsal*. C *bcal*.
160. A, C *sgrub*.
161. A, B, C *btsal*.
162. C *sgrubs*.

(34)/nga la 'jug pa'i rim pa'i lam med de//rang 'byung ye shes dus gcig[163] rdzogs pa'i phyir//ma bgrod rang bzhin bzhag[164] pas phyin par 'gyur/(Chap. 64)

(35)/kye rig pa'i rgyal po sems dpa' rdo rje[165] nyon//don dam nges pa'i[166] lung zhes bstan pa ni//rig pa'i rgyal pos rig gam bstan du med//mi gnas dmigs par bya ba'i yul ma yin//mi rtog rtog las 'das pa'i rang bzhin la[167]//ting 'dzin mi sgom[168] bsam pa'i yul dang bral//'dod pa'i sems med blang ba'i 'bras med de[169]//mi rtog ji bzhin pa ru gnas pa des//lam la ma bgrod sangs rgyas sa ru phyin//rig pa ma sbyangs rang 'byung ye shes rnyed//'phrin[170] las ma btsal rang bzhin lhun gyis grub//dam tshig mi sdom rang bzhin rnam par dag /yul dang dbang po de bzhin nyid du gsal[171]//sangs rgyas sems can gnyis su ma mthong ste//de bzhin nyid du thams cad gcig par mthong//de bzhin nyid la gcig dang du ma med// ma byung ma skyes pa yi snying po la//sgros kyis btags pa'i tha snyad ga la yod/ (Chap. 33)

(36)/gang zhig sangs rgyas yod par mthong ba ni//chos nyid dbyings las sangs rgyas mi rnyed de[172]//sangs rgyas ma lta rang sems bya med rtogs/ (Chap. 15)

(37)/nga ni chos kun rang bzhin yin pa ste//nga yi rang bzhin las ni chos gzhan med//ston pa sku gsum nga yi rang bzhin yin//dus gsum sangs rgyas nga yi rang bzhin yin//byang

---

163. C cig.
164. A, B gzhag.
165. A, B chen po.
166. A pa.
167. B las.
168. A bsgom.
169. A bu med.
170. C phrin.
171. C bsal.
172. A te.

chub sems dpa' nga yi rang bzhin yin//rnal 'byor rnam bzhi nga yi rang bzhin yin//'dod khams gzugs khams gzugs med khams gsum yang//kun byed nga yi rang bzhin bstan pa yin[173]//'byung chen lnga yang nga yi rang bzhin yin//rgyud drug sems can nga yi rang bzhin yin//snang ba thams cad nga yi rang bzhin yin//srid pa thams cad nga yi rang bzhin yin//snod bcud bsdus pa nga yi rang bzhin yin//nga yi rang bzhin las ni gzhan med pas//chos rnams kun gyi[174] rtsa ba nga la[175] 'dus//nga la[176] ma 'dus pa ni gcig kyang med/ (Chap. 11)

(38)/kun byed nga ni kun tu gsang ba'o//nga las byung ba'i sku gsum ston pa la//nga yi rang bzhin rnam gsum mi bstan gsang//nga la gnas pa'i dus gsum sangs rgyas la/[177]/nga yi rang bzhin mi bstan gsang bar bya//nga la 'dus pa'i 'khor tshogs thams cad la//nga yi rang bzhin mi bstan gsang[178] bar bya//nga yis byas pa'i khams gsum sems can la//nga yi rang bzhin mi bstan gsang[179] bar bya/[180]/nga yi rang bzhin ma gsang bstan byas na[181]//sku gsum ston pa[182] nga las 'byung mi 'gyur//sku gsum ston pa nga las ma byung na[183]//bstan[184] gsum theg gsum 'khor gsum[185] tshogs[186] mi 'gyur//bstan gsum theg gsum 'khor gsum[187] ma tshogs[188] na//sangs rgyas chos dang dge 'dun dkon

---

173. C *yi*.
174. C *gyis*.
175. C *las*.
176. C *las*.
177. B inserts /*nga yi rang bzhin sku gsum ston pa la*/.
178. C *bsang*.
179. C *bsang*.
180. A inserts /*nga yi rang bzhin sku gsum ston pa la*/.
181. C *nas*.
182. C *par*.
183. C *nas*.
184. C *stan*.
185. B *phun sum*.
186. A *'tshogs*.

mchog gsum//bla med byang chub kun gyis[189] rig pa med/ /nga las byung ba'i dus gsum sangs rgyas la//nga yi rang bzhin ma gsang[190] bstan 'gyur[191] na//sku gsum ston gsum med pa'i skyon du 'gyur//nga la 'dus pa 'khor gyi tshogs rnams[192] la//nga yi rang bzhin ma gsang bstan gyur[193] na//ston gsum theg pa'i[194] khyad par phyed mi 'gyur//nga yis byas pa'i khams gsum sems can la//nga yi rang bzhin thugs rjes[195] bstan gyur[196] na//ston pa gsum gyi[197] bstan pa'i[198] gnas med 'gyur//ston pa gsum gyi bstan pa'i[199] gnas med na//kun byed nga yis byas pa'i chos rnams la//phun sum tshogs pa zhes su[200] su zhig[201] 'dogs/(Chap. 14)

(39)/de nas byang chub kyi sems kun byed rgyal po des nyid kyi rang bzhin dang/ nyid kyi ngo bo dang/ nyid kyi thugs rje las chos thams cad bkod pa ni/ nyid kyi rang 'byung gi ye shes chen po gcig las/ rang 'byung gi ye shes chen po lnga phyung ba ni 'di lta te/ zhes sdang rang 'byung ye shes chen po dang/ 'dod chags rang 'byung ye shes chen po dang/ gti mug rang 'byung ye shes chen po dang//phrag dog rang 'byung ye shes chen po dang/ nga rgyal rang 'byung ye shes chen po dang/ rang 'byung gi ye shes lnga po des rgyan gyi

---

187. A, B *phun sum.*
188. A *'tshogs.*
189. C *gyi.*
190. C *bsang.*
191. C *'gyur.*
192. A, B *'dus pa'i dus gsum 'khor tshogs.*
193. C *'gyur.*
194. C *pa.*
195. A, B *rje.*
196. A *gyur.*
197. C *gyis.*
198. A, B *pa.*
199. A, B *pa.*
200. A, B *ni.*

rgyu chen po lnga ni phyung/ 'jig cing rten pa'i khams chen po gsum ni bkod de/ rgyan gyi rgyu'i lus lnga gcig tu blangs pa ni 'di lta ste/ rgyan gyi rgyu'i lus sa zhes bya ba'i lus dang/ rgyan gyi rgyu'i lus chu zhes bya ba'i lus dang/ rgyan gyi rgyu'i lus me zhes bya ba'i lus dang/ rgyan gyi rgyu'i lus rlung zhes bya ba'i lus dang/ rgyan gyi rgyu'i lus nam mkha' zhes bya ba'i lus la gcig tu lus thams cad blangs/(Chap. 2)

(40)/rnam par thar pa'i lam ni rnam lnga ste//dus gsum sangs rgyas kun gyi lam du bstan//rang 'byung ye shes lnga yi lam lnga ni/./'dod chags dang ni zhe sdang gti mug dang// nga rgyal dang ni phrag dog rnam lnga ste//rang 'byung ye shes rnam lnga kun gyi lam/(Chap. 3)

(41) /de bzhin nyid ni 'di lta[202] ste//kun byed nga yang de bzhin nyid//ngas byas kun kyang de bzhin nyid//yul drug nga yis byas pa yin//dbang drug nga yi[203] rig pa yin//rnam par shes pa'i tshogs rnams ni//nga yi rang 'byung ye shes yin/ /'byung chen lnga yang rgyu lnga ste//kun[204] gyi rgyu lnga de bzhin nyid//thugs rje rang 'byung ye shes lnga//khams gsum rgyud drug phyung ba yang//de bzhin nyid kyi ngo bor bshad/(Chap. 8)

(42)/des na kun byed rgyal po nga yis ni//nga yi rang bzhin nga yis phyung nas ni//nga la nga yi rang bzhin nga yis[205] bstan//nga las byung ba'i ston pa[206] 'khor rnams la//bstan pa'i lung ni kun byed ngas ma phog /shin tu rnal 'byor kun byed nga yin pas//de la nga yi[207] rang bzhin bstan par bya/ (Chap. 14)

---

201. A, B *yis*.
202. C *blta*.
203. B *yis*.
204. B *rgyan*.
205. C *la*.
206. A, B *pa'i*.
207. C *kun byed*.

Kun byed rgyal po

(43)/sems nyid skye ba[208] med par[209] kun smra zhing//rang bzhin med pa'i don la kun rtsod[210] kyang//skye[211] med mngon du kun[212] gyis rtogs pa med/(Chap. 80)

(44)/ston pa'i ston pa kun byed rgyal po yis/[213]/rnam rtog mtshan ma'i lam la gnas pa'i bar//bsrung dang mi bsrung khyad par gnyis mthong ba[214]//rtsa ba yan lag bcas pa bsrung bar bstan//kye kun byed nga ni ye nas de bzhin nyid//de bzhin nyid la bzung 'dzin med pa'i phyir//chos rnams de ltar gang gis rtogs pa la//bsrung dang mi bsrung 'du shes 'jug pa med/(Chap. 72)

(45)/ji ltar snang ba'i chos rnams ma lus pa[215]//skye[216] med chos kyi dbyings su kun gcig[217] pas//skye med snying po thugs kyi rang bzhin la//sgrib dang[218] mi sgrib[219] khyad par bstan pa med//kye sems dpa' rdo rje legs par sgoms[220] shig /skye med chos kyi dbyings su gcig pa la//sgrib dang mi sgrib spong len gang 'dod pa//dam pa'i snying po'i don dang 'gal bar 'gyur/[. . .]/mkha' ltar rtog spyod 'das la[221] gang gnas pa[222]// sgrib dang mi sgrib byang chub sems su gnas/(Chap. 79)

---

208. C *pa*.
209. A *skye med yin par*.
210. A *brtsod*.
211. C *kye*.
212. C *mngon sum dus*.
213. B inserts /*nga las byung ba'i ston pa sku gsum gyis*/.
214. A *sa*. B *bas*.
215. A *la*.
216. C *kye*.
217. C *cig*.
218. C *pa*.
219. C *bsgrib*.
220. A, C *bsgoms*.
221. B *la ni*.
222. C *pas*.

(46)/dus gsum chos nyid 'gyur ba med pa'i phyir//kun byed rgyal po nga yi dam tshig ni//dus gsum du ni[223] bsrung du med par rtogs[224]//kye chos rnams rtsa ba sems su gcig pa ltar//dam tshig rtsa ba bsrung du med par gcig[225] /de yang rang sems skye med rtogs pa yin/(Chap. 60).

---

223. A, B *kun du*.
224. A, B *ston*.
225. C *cig*.

Index

abhidharma, *see* philosophical studies

accomplished naturally (*lhun gyis grub*), 107; *see also* innate realization, naturally present, spontaneously present

ages (*bskal pa*), 15, 18, 27

antidote (*gnyen po*), 84, 93

anuttarayoga, *see* Higher Tantras

anuyoga (subsequent union), 79n, 117n, 125n

ati, spyi ti, yang ti, 89n

Atiyoga (*shin tu rnal 'byor*), v, 51, 83-84, 117n, 119, 125-26; *see also* Extreme Union, Dzogchen, Great Completeness

awareness (*rig pa*), 27-28, 32, 52 *passim*; *see also* introduction

awareness of spontaneous knowledge (*rang byung ye shes rig pa*), 115

awareness of the present moment (*da lta'i rig pa*), 98

Buddha-nature, 47, 110; *see also* essence of the realized beings

cakra, *see* energy centre

Cakrasaṁvara, 22

caryā (ceremonial), 79n, 117n

cause and effect (*rgyu dang 'bras bu*), 81, 83, 85, 125

clarity (*gsal ba*), 16, 25, 71, 74, 90, 93, 101, 113, 120

clear light (*'od gsal*), 15, 18, 21, 27, 78, 97, 124

commitment (*dam tshig*), 19-20, 22, 35, 75, 82-83, 85, 96, 107, 123

completion process (*rdzogs rim*), 26

conduct (*spyod pa*), 19, 23-24, 28, 30, 85, 96, 98-100, 104-05, 107-08, 111

consciousness (*sems*), 12 *passim*, 76 *passim*; *see also* mind

consciousness series (*sems sde*), 126

creation process (*bskyed rim*), 26

deed of power (*'phrin las*), 83, 85, 96, 107

definitive doctrine (*nges lung*), 83, 106; *see also* provisional doctrine

Dharma (teaching), 76n

dharmakāya, see reality body

dharmamudrā, see seal of the teaching

Diamond Being (rDo rje sems dpa'), 22, 38, 46, 102-03, 126

Diamond Fairy (rDo rje mkha' 'gro), 10, 34

Dzogchen (*rdzogs chen*), 45, 51-53, 81, 107; *see also* Great Completeness, Atiyoga

effort (*rtsol, bya rtsol, rtsol sgrub*), 20, 23, 25, 39, 44, 70-71, 75, 80, 82-83, 85, 91, 94, 98, 100, 102, 119

eleven vehicles (*theg pa bcu gcig*), 89

emanation body (*sprul sku*), 71-72, 74, 89-90, 117n

emptiness and bliss (*bde stong*), 33-34

empty form (*stong gzugs*), 10, 26

empty, emptiness (*stong pa, stong pa nyid*), 15-16, 31, 33-34, 70-71, 74, 90, 93-94, 97, 101, 109, 113, 120, 122

energy centre, 33

enlightened consciousness (*byang chub sems*), 69, 70 *passim*

essence of the realized beings (*bde gshegs snying po*), 89, 109; *see also* Buddha-nature

essence, existence and grace (*rang bzhin, ngo bo, thugs rje*), 71, 118

eternalism, 78n

ethical rules (*'dul ba*), 18, 98

Extreme Union (*shin tu rnal 'byor*), 51, 84, 119; *see also* Atiyoga

feeling of the present moment (*da lta'i shes pa, da lta'i shes rig*), 93, 99-100, 104-05, 110

feeling oneself in the present moment (*da lta rang gi shes pa*), 92, 104, 120

five emotional poisons (*nyon mongs dug lnga*), 115, 118

four initiations, 22

fourth initiation, 35

fruition body (*longs sku, longs spyod rdzogs sku*), 71-72, 89-90, 117n

Garab Dorje, 123

goal (*'bras bu*), 18, 23-24, 30-31, 42, 45, 52, 82, 86, 94, 96, 98-100, 105, 107-08, 111

God of gods (*lha'i lha*), 127

gradual path (*rim gyis pa, rim pa'i lam*), 3, 35, 103

grater vehicle, 117n

Great Completeness (*rdzogs chen, rdzogs pa chen po*), 51, 81, 85, 94; *see also* Dzogchen, Atiyoga

great nail (*gzer chen*), 99-100

Great Seal (*phyag rgya chen po*), 3-4, 10-11, 16-18, 22, 24, 26, 28-30, 32, 35, 38, 40-41, 43, 45-46, 89, 110; *see also* Mahāmudrā

Index

Great Self (*bdag nyid chen po*), 74-76, 124
great thread (*thig chen*), 99
guru-yoga, 22

hearers (*nyan thos*), 78n, 89
hīnayāna, see lesser vehicle
Higher Tantras, 22

innate realization (*lhun gyis grub pa, lhun grub*), 98, 105; see accomplished naturally, naturally present, spontaneously present
instantaneous path (*cig car ba*), 3
intellect (*blo*), 27-28, 35, 43, 106; see also mind
introduction (*ngo sprod*), 74, 77, 90, 92-93, 101-05, 121, 123
I-thought (*sems kyi ngar 'dzin*), 42; see also thought of the I

kalpa, see ages
Karma Lingpa (Kar ma gling pa), 124
karmamudrā, see seal of action
kriyā (ritual action), 79n, 117n
Kunje Gyalpo (Kun byed rgyal po), 76, 124, 126; see also sovereign creator of all

lesser vehicle, 117n
love, 34, 47, 74, 76, 108-09, 114, 125

Mahāmudrā (*phyag rgya chen po*), v, 3, 26, 43, 45; see also Great Seal
mahāyāna, see greater vehicle
mahāyoga (great union), 79n, 117n
Mandāravā, 124
mantra, 17, 23, 51, 83
matrix (*snying po*), 70-72, 75, 80, 96, 100, 107, 122
means and wisdom (*thabs dang shes rab*), 33-34, 108, 120
meditation (*sgom pa*), 3, 23-25, 30, 45, 80, 82, 90, 94, 96, 98-100, 104-05, 107
middle way (*dbu ma*), 78n, 89, 109
mind (*sems, yid, blo*), 17, 27-28, 31-32, 40-41, 83, 91, 98, 110 *passim*; see also intellect

Nālandā, 24
Nāropa, 3, 24
natural liberation (*rang grol*), 74-75, 85, 87, 123; see also self-liberation
natural state (*rnal ma, rang gnas, ngang, rang bzhin, rnal bzhag, rang sa*), 12, 16-18, 25, 29-30, 32, 41, 44-45, 70-71, 75, 81-82, 84, 86-89, 91-92, 101-03, 108, 111-13, 116-19, 123
natural wisdom (*rang 'byung ye shes*), 71n, 72, 74, 118n, 119; see also spontaneous knowledge
naturally present (*lhun grub*), 82, 91; see also accomplished naturally, innate realization, spontaneously present

nihilism, 78n
nine vehicles (*theg pa rim dgu*), 114, 121
nirmāṇakāya, see emanation body
non-action (*bya ba med pa*), 83-85, 87-88, 102

ordinary feeling (*tha mal shes pa*), 89, 104, 110

Padmasambhava, 22, 51, 74, 123
panacea, 46
pāramitā, see perfections
peaceful and wrathful deities (*zhi khro*), 22, 74, 76
perfections (*pha rol phyin pa*), 28
philosophical studies (*mngon pa*), 18, 98
prajñā, 34; *see also* means and wisdom
pratyeakabuddha, see spontaneous victors
preliminary practices, 75
presence (*dran pa*), 44, 102-03, 109
Primordial Buddha (*ye sangs rgyas*), 46-47, 71-72, 88, 125, 127; *see also* Universal Goodness
provisional doctrine (*drang lung*), 80, 83; *see also* definitive doctrine

reality body (*chos sku*), 71-72, 89-90, 97, 101-02, 117n
rig pa, see awareness

saṁbhogakāya, see fruition body
Samantabhadra, *see* Universal Goodness
samaya, *see* commitment
samayamudrā, see seal of commitment
sattvayoga, 125n
seal of action (*las kyi phyag rgya*), 33
seal of commitment, 22
seal of the teaching, 33
secret empowerment (*gsang dbang*), 33; *see also* four initiations
self-aware knowledge (*rang rig ye shes*), 104
self-awareness (*rang rig, rang gi rig pa*), 12, 31, 38, 42-43, 74-75, 82, 90, 97, 101, 104, 112, 121, 123
self-liberation, 43, 109, 123; *see also* natural liberation
self-resplendent (*rang gsal*), 38, 69, 92, 94, 104-05
short path (*gseng lam*), 3, 35
single point (*thig le nyag gcig*), 89, 100, 104
six beings (*rgyud drug, rgyud drug sems can, 'gro ba rigs drug, sems can rigs drug*), 78n, 114-16, 119
source and awareness (*dbyings rig*), 79n
source and knowledge (*dbyings dang ye shes*), 89
source of reality (*chos kyi dbyings*), 73, 89

Index

sovereign creator of all (*kun byed rgyal po*), 70-71, 81-82, 96, 98, 117-19, 122-23; *see also* Kunje Gyalpo

spontaneous knowledge (*rang 'byung ye shes*), 70-71, 89, 92, 94, 96-97, 103-04, 107-08, 111, 113, 118-19, 126; *see also* natural wisdom

spontaneous knowledge of awareness (*rang 'byung rig pa'i ye shes*), 72

spontaneous victors (*rang rgyal*), 78n

spontaneously present (*lhun grub*), 93; *see also* accomplished naturally, innate realization, naturally present, spontaneously present

śrāvaka, *see* hearers

Śrī Siṁha, 121, 123

Sūtra (*mdo*, instructions), 3, 18, 73, 98, 112n

Tantra (*rgyud*, esoteric tradition), 3, 18, 34-35, 51-52, 73, 79, 98, 112n, 117n

third esoteric initiation, 33, 35; *see also* four initiations

thought of the I (*ngar 'dzin rnam rtog*), 92, 101, 124; *see also* I-thought

three bodies (*sku gsum*), 71, 77, 81-83, 90-91, 98, 105, 117; *see also* reality body, fruition body, emanation body

three series of consciousness (*sems sde*), of space (*klong sde*) and of advice (*man ngag sde*), 125

tīrthika, 78n

Tilopa, 3

transcendent knowledge (*shes rab pha rol phyin pa*), 89, 110

transmigration and liberation (*'khor 'das*), 47, 76-77, 80-81, 89, 92, 98, 108, 110-12, 114-16, 118, 125, 127

true nature of consciousness (*sems kyi rang bzhin, sems nyid*), 16, 25, 70, 89-90, 92-94, 113, 121, 124

true nature of reality (*chos nyid, dngos po'i gnas lugs, chos kyi dbyings*), 17, 72, 84, 90, 94, 96, 102, 110, 112, 122

true nature of self-aware consciousness (*rang rig sems nyid*), 104-05

ubhaya (twofold), 79n, 117n

Uḍḍiyāna, 51, 74, 123

unaltered (*ma bcos*), 10-11, 14-15, 71-72, 75, 82, 84, 92, 95, 98, 102, 104, 111

unborn (*skye ba med pa, mi skye, ma skyes*), 29, 72-73, 76, 81, 94, 96-97, 100, 102, 107, 116, 122-23

universal base (*kun gzhi*), 29, 44, 89, 92, 110

Universal Goodness (Kun tu bzang po), 47, 71, 88, 125; *see* Primordial Buddha

upāya, 34; *see also* means and wisdom

utpannakrama, see completion process

utpattikrama, see creation process

Vajraḍākinī, *see* Diamond Fairy

Vajrasattva, *see* Diamond Being

vase empowerment *(bum dbang)*, 22; *see* four initiations

view *(lta ba)*, 23, 30, 80, 82-85, 94, 96, 98-100, 104-05, 107-08

vinaya, see ethical rules

virtue and vice *(dge sdig)*, 14, 21, 122

Wheel of Time (Kālacakra), 46

Yeshe Tsogyal, 124

yoga, 79n, 117n